Penguin Health

Chiropractic for Everyone

Anthea Courtenay has been working as a [...] and translator for sixteen years. She has published some forty short stories and translated a number of children's history books from their original French. Her articles have been published in a great many magazines and newspapers, including *Good House-keeping*, *Woman's Journal*, the *Guardian* and the *Sunday Express* magazine.

She has always been interested in alternative medicine, healing and the mind–body relationship, and recently these subjects have become a specialist area of her work. She has contributed features on them to *Time Out*, *Fitness*, the *Journal of Alternative Medicine* and *Woman*, among others. She has also researched six audio tapes on self-healing for the healer Matthew Manning, the topics being Depression, Addiction, Arthritis, Insomnia, Allergies and Eyesight. She has written and recorded 'Just Imagine', an audio tape for children on creative relaxation.

ANTHEA COURTENAY

CHIROPRACTIC FOR EVERYONE

YOUR SPINE AND YOUR HEALTH

PENGUIN BOOKS

Penguin Books Ltd, Harmondsworth, Middlesex, England
Viking Penguin Inc., 40 West 23rd Street, New York, New York 10010, U.S.A.
Penguin Books Australia Ltd, Ringwood, Victoria, Australia
Penguin Books Canada Limited, 2801 John Street, Markham, Ontario, Canada L3R 1B4
Penguin Books (N.Z.) Ltd, 182–190 Wairau Road, Auckland 10, New Zealand

First published 1987

Copyright © Anthea Courtenay, 1987
Illustrations by David Gifford
All rights reserved

Made and printed in Great Britain by
Richard Clay Ltd, Bungay, Suffolk
Typeset in 11/13 Plantin

Except in the United States of America, this book is sold subject
to the condition that it shall not, by way of trade or otherwise, be lent,
re-sold, hired out, or otherwise circulated without the
publisher's prior consent in any form of binding or cover other than
that in which it is published and without a similar condition
including this condition being imposed on the subsequent purchaser

CONTENTS

ACKNOWLEDGEMENTS

I should like to express my grateful thanks for all the time, information and help given to me by the numerous chiropractors, patients, doctors and surgeons whose knowledge and experience have been essential to the writing of this book. In particular my thanks to George Walker and Susan Moore of the British Chiropractic Association, to Stanley Harding and Bronwen Herbertson of the Institute of Pure Chiropractic for their continuing help, and to James Rousseau and Alison Gordon-Creed for their caring attention to my own back.

Note

A number of chiropractors, doctors and patients have kindly given me permission to use their names in describing their views and case histories, and I have taken the opportunity to do so wherever possible rather than confront the reader with an accumulation of anonymous quotations. Neither I nor the practitioners concerned would wish these references to be regarded as an advertisement for their particular services. The number of chiropractors I have been able to talk with personally has obviously been limited, and those who are named in these pages have agreed to be quoted as representatives of a profession of which they are proud.

A.C.

Illustrations

Permission to use the illustrations on the following pages is gratefully acknowledged:
page 10: Wellcome Institute Library, London; *pages 11 and 21:* Chiropractic; *pages 35, 37 and 46:* Anglo-European College of Chiropractic Ltd; *page 58:* E. Bridge (artist); *pages 62, 63 and 175:* Institute of Pure Chiropractic; *pages 75 and 77:* British Chiropractic Association; *pages 88, 92, 93, 206 and 207: from The Back: Relief from Pain* by Dr Alan Stoddard (1979), Martin Dunitz; *pages 197 and 199:* from *Medicine Men* by John Lloyd Fraser (1981), Thames Methuen; *page 201: Talkback* (April 1986), Back Pain Association.
    The remainder of the illustrations have been drawn by David Gifford.

PART ONE

THE DEVELOPMENT OF CHIROPRACTIC

CHAPTER ONE

THE BIRTH OF AN ART

I am the originator, the Fountain Head ... I have answered the
time-worn question – what is life?

D. D. Palmer

Manipulating the human spine is one of the oldest and most
widespread therapies in the world. The earliest written
account of it has been found in a Chinese document, the
Kong Fou, dated around 2700 B.C.; manipulative therapies
were practised throughout the civilizations of the ancient
world, including ancient Greece. The early fathers of medicine, the Greek physicians Hippocrates and Galen, practised spinal manipulation and preached the importance of
the spine in relation to bodily health. As well as manual
adjustment, Hippocrates is credited with inventing a rather
fearsome-looking mechanical device for stretching the
spine by traction; he also recommended sitting on patients,
if necessary, or shaking them while they were hanging from
ladders.

During the Dark Ages after the fall of Rome in A.D. 476,
hundreds of libraries and records were destroyed, and
health care deteriorated into superstition and magic. In a
Europe where health was constantly endangered by
plagues, physicians hesitated to lay their hands on patients
who might contaminate them. Manipulative techniques
were carried on among country people by naturally gifted
bone-setters (there are still some today), setting the scene

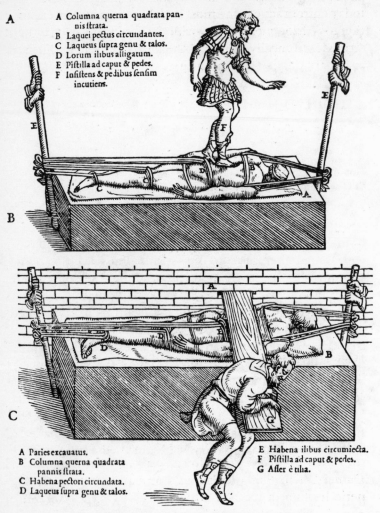

A
A Columna querna quadrata pan-
  nis ſtrata.
B Laquei pectus circundantes.
C Laqueus ſupra genu & talos.
D Lorum ilibus alligatum.
E Piſtilla ad caput & pedes.
F Inſiſtens & pedibus ſenſim
  incutiens.

B

C
A Paries excauatus.
B Columna querna quadrata
  pannis ſtrata.
C Habena pectori circundata.
D Laqueus ſupra genu & talos.

E Habena ilibus circumiecta.
F Piſtilla ad caput & pedes.
G Aſſer è tilia.

Ancient methods of spinal manipulation and traction

for the present divide between orthodox medicine and the
positioning of chiropractic and osteopathy as 'alternative'
therapies. These techniques were initially regarded by
medicine with distrust and disbelief, which in the case of

chiropractic continued in America for many decades. Yet today chiropractic is the most widely recognized alternative therapy throughout the world. It has been a long, hard struggle, ironically rendered the harder by the enthusiasm and individuality of its pioneers.

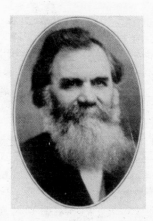

Daniel David Palmer (1845–1913), 'the Discoverer'

Daniel David Palmer

The history of chiropractic began on a September day in 1895 when Harvey Lillard, the black caretaker of a block in the town of Davenport, Iowa, walked into the office of Daniel David Palmer. Palmer was a practitioner of magnetic healing, a method which involved the laying on of hands; a short, thickset fifty-year-old, his mane of greying hair and heavy beard enhanced a compelling personality. Lillard was extremely deaf – too deaf to hear the horse-drawn traffic four floors below – and Palmer began questioning him about his condition. Seventeen years before, Lillard told him, he had been working in a stooped position when he felt something give in his back; almost immediately he lost his hearing. Palmer tried giving him magnetic treatment, with no effect. Examining Lillard's spine, he found a painful and prominent vertebra in the upper part of the back. Yes, said Lillard, that was the place that had hurt when he lost his hearing. Palmer asked him to lie face downwards on his treatment table, and exerted an energetic manual thrust on the vertebra in question. Shortly afterwards, Lillard announced that he was beginning to hear again. The first chiropractic adjustment had been made.

Palmer later wrote that the event was no accident; the adjustment 'was accomplished with an object in view, and the result expected was obtained. There was nothing crude about this adjustment; it was specific.' He had in fact been working towards it for some years.

A colourful, eccentric non-conformist, Palmer had already followed a varied career. He was born in 1845, 'way out West' in the small Canadian town of Port Perry near Toronto, of Scotch and Irish ancestry on his mother's side, English and German on his father's. His father was a shoemaker and later a grocer, who also served as community schoolmaster and postmaster. Times were hard, and in 1865 Daniel left home with his brother to seek for better opportunities in the United States. In 1866 he settled in New Boston, Illinois, where he became a successful beekeeper. In 1876 he married his housekeeper and they moved to the delightfully named What Cheer, Iowa, where he ran a grocery store and fathered three children. In the course of his career he also was a village schoolmaster, and made and lost money in several small commercial ventures.

In 1885, following his wife's death, Palmer moved to Davenport, Iowa, where he set up his practice in magnetic healing, a skill he had learned from Paul Caster, an internationally known practitioner. Magnetic healing – which derived from the 'magnetism' developed by the eighteenth-century Austrian Franz Mesmer – was just one fringe or natural therapy enjoying popularity in the USA in those times. Medicine, particularly in the West and Midwest, was far from satisfactory. There were few doctors, and many of those were only half trained; medical treatment consisted of purges, blood-letting and a heavy-handed use of such drugs as were available. (There was also a lively non-medical trade in the peddling of spurious elixirs based largely on alcohol.)

On the east coast, as in Europe, medicine was progressing towards its present scientific basis. Pasteur had established his theory of germs in the 1860s, and the tubercle bacillus was identified in the 1880s. Joseph Lister was working obsessively on establishing the case for antiseptic surgery. But in the meantime in America dissatisfaction with medical methods and the sheer lack of trained doctors in rural areas had encouraged throughout the nineteenth century a general interest in natural healing methods, including diet, herbs, exercise, electricity, purges, bone-setting, religious healing, magnetic healing, sunshine, homoeopathy and mineral baths. This setting provided a fertile seedbed for the growth of two new major schools: osteopathy and chiropractic.

Osteopathy came first. In 1864 the three children of a country doctor, Andrew Taylor Still, died of spinal meningitis, a tragedy which crystallized Still's disillusionment with orthodox medicine. The son of a Methodist preacher and hand healer, Still had studied engineering as well as training briefly in medicine; he developed the theory that many ailments stemmed from distortions or malfunctions in the structure of the body. (He declared in his later writings that this had been revealed to him by God.)

His theory was that the body cannot function properly unless it is structurally sound: if the structure is made sound, the body's own 'life force' will take over to restore health. His method depended on what he called 'the rule of the artery'. When blood circulates normally, 'disease cannot develop, because our blood is capable of manufacturing all the necessary substance to maintain natural immunity against disease'. When blood becomes static, it goes 'sour' and illness follows. Strains or dislocations in the spine impede the proper flow of the 'fluids of life'; therefore treating structural and mechanical spinal derangements or 'lesions' liberates and purifies the bloodstream, restoring normal body function. Although he made his discovery in 1874, Still did not set up his American School of Osteopathy, at Kirksville in Missouri, until 1892 – three years before Palmer adjusted Harvey Lillard's back.

D. D. Palmer, meanwhile, was on his own quest for the cause of disease. He, too, had observed the failures of medicine. Drugs were not the answer: 'Why drug the entire body,' he was to ask, 'when only one organ is sick?' Although he seems to have been successful as a healer he felt that he was only treating effects; he believed that all ill-health stemmed from a fundamental cause, and could only be satisfactorily treated when that cause had been found. Like Still – and like many others before him, including Hippocrates – he believed that the body had its own natural healing forces. When an organ was sick, something must be impeding the flow of these forces: somewhere between brain and organ there was a 'damming backward, with a starving supply forward'.

Later on, osteopaths were to accuse chiropractic of being 'a pure steal'. Palmer must certainly have been aware of Still's work; although his son later denied that he had ever been near Kirksville, it was only a day's journey away, and with his interest in healing it would have been curious had he not paid it a visit. However, while there are many similarities between osteopathy and chiropractic there were and are differences. In his book *The Chiropractor* (1914), D. D. Palmer was to instruct: 'Don't do anything as an osteopath does.' (The two schools have followed quite different paths in England and America, as will be seen.)

Still was not the only person to relate the health of the spine to general health, and certainly not the first. Hippocrates, whom Palmer admired, had written in the fourth century B.C., 'Get knowledge of the spine, for this is the requisite for many diseases', while Galen, the Greek 'prince of physicians', had told his students, 'Look to the nervous system as the key to maximum health.' In the nineteenth century several medical doctors and scientists were studying both the spine and the nervous system. In 1843 J. Evans Riadore, a physician, had written a book called *Irritation of the Spinal Nerves* in which he related irritation of the spinal nerve roots to a deficient supply of nervous energy or blood, leading to organic disease; and in 1894 the English physician Sir William Gowers stated that 'function depends upon the release of force – nerve force'. Physicians had already tried using leeches and cauteries on the spine in attempts to treat disease in organs on parallel body segments.

Palmer had had no formal education but he was intelligent, intuitive, and energetically dedicated to his self-imposed quest. He set himself to study the available literature, to question doctors, and to teach himself anatomy and physiology, and was also to claim that he had obtained the explanation of certain physical phenomena through divine inspiration. He wrote later: 'One question was always uppermost in my mind in my search for the Cause of Disease. I desired to know why one person was ailing and his associate working in the same shop at the same bench was not. This question was answered in September, 1895, with my first chiropractic adjustment.' If the vertebrae of the spine were misaligned, he reasoned, this must affect the human nervous system; adjust the spine and healing will follow.

With a regular clientele visiting him for magnetic healing, he had ample opportunity to test his theories further. Shortly afterwards he was visited by a patient whose heart trouble was not responding to orthodox medical treatment. Palmer examined his spine and, as he wrote later, 'found a displaced vertebra pressing against the nerves which innervate the heart'. He adjusted the vertebra and the patient's condition immediately began to improve. 'Then I began to clearly reason, if two diseases so dissimilar as deafness and heart trouble came from a spinal impingement, causing a pressure upon nerves, were not other diseases due to a similar cause?'

It is understandable that he should come to such a conclusion; it is also curious that Palmer's first two chiropractic cases were of types that today are scarcely obvious candidates for spinal manipulation. But success in an increasing number of cases, together with his observation that displaced vertebrae were the rule rather than the exception in the sick, seemed to prove Palmer's theory: the basis of all disease lay in the spine; misaligned or maladjusted vertebrae restricted nerves, and this interference with the flow of nervous impulses prevented the body's life force from carrying out healing. Ninety-five per cent of all diseases were caused by misaligned vertebrae restricting nerve flow; relieving the pressure upon these nerves by adjustment would restore normal health.

Among his patients was the Reverend Samuel Weed; Palmer had treated his daughter's sprained ankle with magnetic healing and was treating Weed himself for TB of the lungs, sciatic rheumatism and dropsy (the reverend gentleman's life force seems to have been in pretty poor shape). Palmer asked him to name his new treatment. Did he know of a Greek word for 'done by hand'? Weed came up with *cheiro praktikos*, and from this the word 'chiropractic' was coined.

Palmer knew perfectly well that people had been adjusting vertebrae for the relief of disease for thousands of years. His system, however, was new, and this he stressed in no uncertain terms. He was to write:

I am the originator, the Fountain Head of the essential principle that disease is the result of too much or not enough functionating. I created the art of adjusting vertebrae, using the spinous and transverse processes* as levers, and named the mental act of accumulating knowledge, the cumulative function, corresponding to the physical vegetative function – growth of intellectual and physical – together, with the science, art and philosophy – Chiropractic ... It was I who combined the science and art and developed the principles thereof. I have answered the time-worn question – what is life?

A Proliferation of Schools

Over the years, D. D. Palmer and his followers refined and revised his theories and practice of chiropractic. A specific terminology was introduced: displacements in the spine came to be called 'subluxations'; the concept of the life force in the individual was interpreted in Palmer terms as 'Innate Intelligence' which was linked to a creative 'Universal Intelligence'. This philosophy was important to Palmer: while happy to blow his own trumpet, he stressed the moral and religious duties of the chiropractor. 'Chiropractic science includes biology – the science of life – in this world, and the recognition of a spiritual existence in the next ...' The basic principle remained the same: 'Displacement of any part of the skeletal frame may press against nerves, which are the channels of communication, intensifying or decreasing their carrying capacity, creating either too much or not enough functioning, an aberration known as disease ...' Spinal subluxations could produce a wide range of symptoms – deafness and heart disease, headaches, digestive disorders, skin problems, let alone backache. No need for drugs; no point in treating symptoms;

*Sections of the facet joints of the spine. See page 87.

simply find the subluxation, correct it, and healing will take place.

It is not surprising that Palmer incurred the enmity of a medical profession which was increasingly viewing health from a mechanistic viewpoint, regarding disease as a happening visited on patients through external agencies such as germs – a theory that Palmer rejected. Yet his early students included medical doctors; one of them, J. S. Riley, M.D., Ph.D., wrote in 1925: 'Some of his cures seemed like miracles, and while we had studied medicine, osteopathy, magnetic healing, mental science, etc., we saw chiropractic doing a work that all the others combined could not do . . .' Chiropractic patients in those days – as is still often the case today – tended to be those with whom conventional medical treatment had failed.

Within a year of his discovery D. D. Palmer began teaching a few students in the building where he had his office, under the name of Dr Palmer's School and Cure. Two years later, in 1897, the Palmer School of Chiropractic offered a six-month course; it had one student in 1898 and a dozen by 1903. In those early days Palmer must have been, briefly, a happy man. For there were plenty of troubles in store – from doctors, osteopaths, rival colleagues, and from his own son, Bartlett Joshua, who graduated from the school (then the Palmer Institute and Chiropractic Infirmary) in 1902 at the age of twenty-one.

Another early student with whom both he and his son B.J. later had disagreements was Willard Carver, a lawyer whose specialization in negligence work had aroused an interest in anatomy and physiology. In the history of chiropractic these three are known as the 'trinity of giants': D.D. was the Founder, B.J. the Developer, and Carver titled himself the Constructor. He made valuable contributions to the development of chiropractic; he recognized that the 'nerve flow' could be impeded in other parts of the body as well as the spine, and made the important observation that if the spine is distorted at one level the body's attempt to compensate will produce distortions at others; he also stressed the importance of correct posture.

Carver founded and ran four chiropractic schools and others were springing up. Palmer founded the Portland College of Chiropractic in partnership with a surgeon and a homoeopath, and in 1907 the Palmer–Gregory School of Chiropractic with a medical doctor, Alva Gregory, in Oklahoma City, then within Indian territory; Gregory had studied at one of Carver's colleges there. Meanwhile in 1904 Palmer had handed over the original and rapidly expanding Davenport school to his son B.J., who had expressed dissatisfaction with his father's management. As students graduated they began setting up small schools of their own, often introducing their own ideas and variations.

Opposition

Although the early chiropractic students included a fair sprinkling of osteopaths, chiropractic was to receive a lot of opposition from osteopathy. Both groups had started mainly with patients who could not afford expensive medical treatment or who lived in districts where doctors were few and far between. By the 1900s both were well established, and were attracting observers and students from overseas. As time went by, osteopaths began to collect a more fashionable clientele, founding medical schools and allying themselves with the medical profession. The doctors, meanwhile, in Brian Inglis's words, 'by this time organized and better aware of the threat to their livelihood, began to assail [chiropractors] with a systematic virulence unequalled in the annals even of the medical profession'.

In the 1880s the medical profession had instigated the Medical Practice Acts, prohibiting non-medical persons from practising medicine without a licence. In 1906 D. D. Palmer was jailed under these Acts. It was a bad year for him all round. After handing the school over to B.J. he had adopted a travelling life, practising and proselytizing throughout the West. In 1906 the ambitious young B.J. published a book on chiropractic (he had written four more by 1910), which D.D. regarded as anatomically and physiologically erroneous; B.J. had also given himself the title of Developer of chiropractic, and granted himself the advanced degree of Ph.C. D.D. responded with his own book, *The Science, Art and Philosophy of Chiropractic*; it, too, has been criticized for its anatomical and physiological inaccuracies, although one writer comments that his writings 'remain remarkable considering that he was self-taught in these sciences'.*

The ageing D.D. was becoming increasingly difficult, and that same year was fraught with disputes with his associates, including Willard Carver, who accused him of over-ambition. In 1910 he quarrelled with Gregory, and the Palmer–Gregory School broke up. In 1911 he returned to Davenport and made a further attempt at working with his son at the Palmer School of Chiropractic; it failed. D.D. then set up a rival school, the Universal Chiropractic College, two blocks away; again, he quarrelled with his partners. He returned to California for a year, and in October 1913 he died in Los Angeles, three months after visiting Davenport to attend the Palmer School's Lyceum and Homecoming.

Few accounts of the Palmers' lives mention the full circumstances of D.D.'s death. At the time he was suffering from the after-effects of an accident that had occurred during his last visit to Davenport, when he was hit by a car in the school parade. 'The car was driven by B.J.,' writes Gibbons,† 'and largely unsubstantiated charges of patricide would linger for years.'

*Russell W. Gibbons, in Scott Haldemann (ed.), *Modern Developments in the Principles and Practice of Chiropractic*, New York, 1979.
†op. cit.

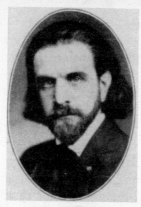

Bartlett Joshua Palmer (1881–1961), 'the Developer'

B. J. Palmer

The Dallasty-like element in the early history of chiropractic, with its colourful characters, and family and professional rivalries, should not blind us to the fact that the focus of all this was a system of healing, of caring for the sick and nurturing the healthy, which was doing a large number of people a great deal of good. It is one of the paradoxes of human creativity that the prophets, healers and gurus who have a genuine truth to offer are often afflicted by oversized egos and touchy personalities.

Bartlett Joshua Palmer, born in 1881, seems to have been even more of a paradox in this respect than his father. He was ambitious, domineering, a self-styled genius who could brook no opposition. He made a striking figure, with his long flowing hair and white linen suits worn with a black silk bow tie. His interests were not limited to chiropractic; he started the second commercial broadcasting station in the USA (all the better for advertising chiropractic, of course).

In 1906 B.J. and his wife Mabel, who also practised and taught chiropractic, moved to the first of a series of bigger premises in the district where the large campus of the

Palmer College stands today. Early students sat on crates in basement classrooms which were damp with seeping water after heavy rainfalls. Nevertheless the school flourished. By 1915 enrolments were over 800; in 1918 there were 1,862 students, drawn from all walks of life and from various professions, including some medical doctors and osteopaths. By now the curriculum included anatomy, physiology, symptomatology, pathology and diagnosis, toxicology, obstetrics and dissection, as well as the science and philosophy of chiropractic.

Although self-educated like his father, B.J. worked hard to give the profession a scientific basis, and a major contribution was his introduction of X-ray equipment to the school as early as 1909. X-rays had been discovered by Roentgen in Germany in the same year that D. D. Palmer adjusted Harvey Lillard's spine; since 1909 they have formed an integral part of chiropractic diagnosis and treatment – marking one major difference between chiropractic and osteopathy. By 1910 the school had collected a library of several hundred glass negatives of the spine which were used for research and teaching. B.J. also assembled the world's largest osteological museum.

B.J.'s greatest ambition was 'to see the chiropractic principle and practice perpetuate itself in its purity for posterity, unfettered and unshackled by antipodal restrictions, legal or otherwise, so that the greatest number of sick under chiropractic care may get well in the quickest possible time'.

The 'antipodal restrictions' were the Medical Practice Acts under which thousands of chiropractors were prosecuted and imprisoned between the two World Wars, often by means of agents paid by doctors to pretend to be patients, in order to accuse chiropractors of performing medical services. The state of Kansas granted legal recognition to chiropractic as early as 1913, but elsewhere the persecution continued. In 1921 in California 450 chiropractors, convicted of practising medicine without a licence, were given the alternative of paying a fine or going to jail. They all chose to go to jail.

The effect was to arouse public sympathy; newspaper offices were bombarded with letters of protest, not only defending chiropractors but also blaming organized medicine for putting up 'decoy evidence' against them. In the first half of this century the American medical profession, though far from being beyond criticism itself, seems to have been particularly jealous of its status. Not only were chiropractors claiming cures which were regarded as medical impossibilities, their patients were pleased with their treatment and were paying less for it than doctors were charging. And they were advertising their services in a Barnum-like fashion which must have been particularly annoying. The printing presses of the Davenport school churned out millions of tracts; B.J. published more than thirty-five books, and promoted chiropractic as the cure for all ills.

In 1924 B.J. created a rift within his own profession. He had invented a technique, vividly entitled 'Hole In One', in which only the first or second cervical vertebra (at the top of the neck) was adjusted. Innate Intelligence, according to B.J., was centred in the brain; the first and second cervical vertebrae therefore occupied 'the vital intermediate space between brain and body' which, if obstructed, resulted in 'starvation of forces or energies made for the body, but not reaching the body'. (All of which sounds extremely quaint; yet, as we shall see, subluxations in the neck do seem responsible for a variety of ills.) B.J. had also invented, in collaboration with Dr Dossa D. Evins of the Palmer School faculty, a diagnostic tool called a neurocalometer, a heat-sensing device whose purpose was to locate temperature-differential areas along the spine, which were supposed to correlate with subluxations.* In a talk at the Davenport

---

*Although some chiropractors still use neurocalometers, they have not been shown to be a reliable diagnostic guide.

school entitled 'The Hour has Struck', B.J. told his audience of thousands that no chiropractor could practise without a neurocalometer, and that any chiropractor not using this with the HIO technique was incapable of practising honestly. He lost the support of a large number of chiropractors, and after this his influence began to wane.

There were further divisions in the profession between the 'straights', who believed in practising chiropractic alone, and the 'mixers', who saw value in including other therapies where appropriate, such as naturopathy or homoeopathy. Two main schools developed: the International Chiropractors Association (ICA), founded by the 'straights' in Davenport in 1926, and the National (now American) Chiropractic Association (NCA), founded in 1930 by the 'mixers'. Some chiropractors, too, were tempted to follow the osteopaths, who in America had become virtually indistinguishable from doctors, but the profession succeeded in keeping its identity as a drug-free, natural method of healing. Both the ICA and the NCA referred to doctors those cases that lay beyond their scope of treatment.

Despite the controversies and divisions, chiropractic continued to spread and by 1931 thirty-nine American states had granted legal recognition to doctors of chiropractic. It was a curious situation. Throughout the inter-war years chiropractors were being jailed on the one hand, and on the other were setting up clinics and hospitals. Though a number of 'fly by night' schools continued to come and go, doing no good at all in the battle against orthodoxy, training in the main schools was vastly improved by the introduction of medical doctors on the staff and medical methods of diagnosis.

B.J. remained active, fascinated by both science and his own theories. In 1935 he produced an instrument for reading brain waves and their conduction through the spinal cord. In the same year he established a research clinic in the school, where he received the seriously ill; it had a full medical and nursing staff, a diagnostic laboratory and physical medicine section. He also operated a chiropractic facility for mental patients at the Clear View Sanitarium. He continued at the same time to preach the importance of Innate Intelligence, and in the 1950s was lecturing on Innate Intelligence and the spiritual significance of sex and phallicism (he had a rare collection of phallic symbols). He died in 1961.

'He was Elbert Hubbard, Titus Oates, Baron Munchausen and P. T. Barnum all rolled into one,' writes Russell Grant, 'yet to his research clinic at midcentury would come "hopeless" and terminal cases – some on referral from the Mayo and Cleveland clinics – to leave apparently cured ... Controversial and colorful, he outraged his detractors in both medicine and chiropractic as much with this style as with his propositions, yet provided an environment for legitimate spinal research and development.'

CHAPTER TWO

CHIROPRACTIC ROUND THE WORLD

Given its somewhat eccentric beginnings, it is quite remarkable that, after medicine and dentistry, chiropractic is
the most widely practised therapy in the world. Its history
almost everywhere has been one of medical opposition con-
trasting with public support; and it is not only popular with
patients, but has been legally recognized by many governments. For although the early claims that it could cure just
about everything have been largely (though not totally)
dropped, it has been shown to provide a safe, drug-free
therapy that is effective with a wide range of musculo-
skeletal disorders, and often improves other conditions.

Over the last century, chiropractic has grown up; there
have been changes in both theory and practice. Techniques
have been refined and new ones introduced; educational
standards have improved and there is greater understanding of the anatomy and function of the nervous system in
both chiropractic and medical circles (though there is still
much to be learned). Below is a brief overview of its development up to 1986; further changes are more than likely
before this book is published.

United States of America

28,553* registered chiropractors (1983). Since 1971 chiropractors have been licensed in all fifty states as primary
health-care providers – that is, they are legally recognized
as providing an alternative medical service to general practice. All states reimburse for the chiropractic treatment of

*Most of the figures in this section have been taken from the *Facts Bulletin* prepared in 1983 by the World Health Development Committee of the International
Chiropractic Association.

industrial accidents and injuries under their workmen's compensation plans. Over three-fifths of the states require inclusion of chiropractic services under all commercial health and accident policies written in those states, and Medicare provides reimbursement for chiropractic treatment.

Chiropractic expanded particularly rapidly after the Second World War, although prosecutions continued into the 1960s, largely at the instigation of the medical profession and often amid public protest. In 1965 in Louisiana, where chiropractic was still unlicensed, half the state's chiropractors were brought before the courts charged with illegally practising medicine; however, the US Court of Appeals, Fifth Circuit, found in their favour. A British chiropractor who trained in America recalls meeting there a chiropractor who had two practices – one in New York City, and one in the prison where he spent regular involuntary periods.

In addition to its effectiveness in treating musculo-skeletal disorders, there are several reasons for chiropractic's survival and success in the United States. One is that chiropractors are the experts in spinal manipulation, since osteopaths have joined mainstream medicine – there are even osteopathic surgeons. Another is the increasing specialization of medicine, which has led to a distrust of doctors, and a diminishing number of GPs; chiropractors have replaced them as family practitioners, though very few of them prescribe drugs (some have taken an additional medical degree in order to do so). Also in their favour is the increasing cost of orthodox medicine in the States – and increasing dissatisfaction with its results. Chiropractic provides a cheaper and often a more effective alternative. For example, in 1960 the Florida Industrial Commission reported on tests carried out on 20,000 cases of back trouble: cases handled by doctors cost over 25 per cent more, compensation costs were over 300 per cent more, and loss of working time under medical treatment was around 300 per cent greater.

Ever since the 1930s chiropractic has been putting its educational house in order. Since the inception of the Council on Chiropractic Education (CCE), which is recognized by the US Department of Health Education and Welfare as the accrediting body for chiropractic colleges, many of the smaller colleges have been done away with and educational curricula standardized. Eleven of the fifteen chiropractic colleges today are accredited by the American CCE, requiring a minimum of six years' study to qualify. Many colleges, like the National College, are described as educating physicians who use chiropractic methods; entrance qualifications and academic teaching are similar to those in medical schools, except that nutrition is taught rather than pharmacology. The Doctor of Chiropractic degree has the same standing as a medical degree, and American chiropractors are entitled to call themselves doctors.

The distinction between 'straights' and 'mixers' has survived. Members of the American Chiropractors Association (ACA) regard themselves as holistic physicians rather than spinal specialists. They incorporate into their treatment other therapies, particularly nutrition and mineral and vitamin supplementation; many of them have been forerunners in this field, as well as in the application of Applied Kinesiology (see page 47).

There is still some conflict between the chiropractic and medical professions, exacerbated by the way in which American chiropractors advertise their services and claim to treat serious conditions. However, the gap between the two is narrowing; younger doctors are more open-minded than the dwindling membership of the American Medical Association.

Canada

2,600 registered chiropractors (1983). Chiropractors are

licensed in all provinces except Newfoundland, with legislation varying in different provinces. In most, workers'
compensation benefits are available for chiropractic treatment, without referral by a medical practitioner. Most
medical benefit schemes include chiropractic. The Canadian
Council of Chiropractic Education is affiliated to the
American CCE.

Other Countries of the American Continent

There are a few chiropractors in Chile, Ecuador, Panama
and the British Virgin Islands, and around forty in Mexico.

Australia

1,100 registered chiropractors (1983). Legal registration
was introduced in 1978 as a result of public support and in
spite of medical opposition. In 1974 the Ministry of Health
appointed a committee to review the evidence, and its findings included independent studies carried out by university
research teams. The committee concluded that chiropractic, while not a complete system of therapy, filled an important gap in health care.

Chiropractic is now included under various government-
funded health plans, including most state Workers' Compensation Acts and state no-fault accident plans, but is not
covered under federal reimbursement plans. A five-year
chiropractic degree programme is offered at the Phillip
Institute of Technology, accredited by the Australian
Council for Chiropractic Education; there is also a non-
accredited two-year postgraduate course run by the Sydney
College of Chiropractic, requiring a B.S. degree in anatomy
for admission.

New Zealand

100 registered chiropractors (1983). Chiropractic was
introduced to New Zealand in 1911 and the New Zealand
Chiropractors Association was incorporated in 1920.

Chiropractors have been registered since 1960, and partial federal reimbursement for treatment is now available under medical referral.

In 1979 a major Commission of Inquiry was set up as a direct result of a petition signed by 97,000 people calling for reimbursement for chiropractic under the government's health plans. It concluded that medical opposition to chiropractic (which in New Zealand has been described as 'vehement and unbending') was largely based on ignorance and misunderstanding. This partly stems from the fact that many New Zealand chiropractors trained in America, and an American-style zeal in publicizing their skills was noted by the Commission with disapproval. However, the therapy itself emerged with flying colours: the Commission concluded that chiropractic is safe, that chiropractors are the only health practitioners necessarily equipped by their education and training to carry it out, and that there should be no impediment to full professional cooperation between chiropractors and medical practitioners. The New Zealand Medical Association, still virulently anti-chiropractic, rejected the report on the grounds that in recommending doctors to refer patients to chiropractors it was requiring them to behave unethically. Despite this, a law registering chiropractors as medical auxiliaries in the manner of physiotherapists was passed in 1983.

The Far East

In 1983 there were fifty chiropractors in Japan, thirteen in Hong Kong, and two in India.

The Middle East

There are a few chiropractors in Egypt, Israel and Cyprus.

South Africa

105 registered chiropractors (1983). Chiropractic is a popular therapy in South Africa, despite the absence of a train-

ing school. In 1971, 176 chiropractors and students were registered, but a Chiropractic Act limited the profession to those then practising or studying to practise it. This ban was lifted in 1984, so new graduates are now able to register. Legislation has been proposed, and the South African Registration Board recognizes the Anglo-European College of Chiropractic in England.

Zimbabwe, Kenya and the Congo

There is a sprinkling of chiropractors in these countries.

Europe

Total number difficult to estimate; approximately 1,000 chiropractors in the European Chiropractors Union (1986).

While chiropractic began in America as a complete system of health care and has largely continued in this direction, legal and other restrictions have encouraged European chiropractors, particularly those in Britain, to become specialists in spinal and joint problems. Apart from Britain, chiropractic is much better known throughout Europe than osteopathy, which is non-existent in some countries. Legislation on alternative therapies varies from country to country, and the over-all picture illustrates the general confusion about their value. However, the European Chiropractors Union (ECU), formed in 1932 as an umbrella for various national chiropractors' associations, at least ensures some cohesiveness among its members.

The ECU has worked hard to improve educational standards and more recently to deal with the issues raised by EEC legislation: for example, an EEC directive on ionizing radiation was originally couched in such a way that it would have restricted the use of X-rays to medical doctors and dentists; the British Chiropractic Association (BCA), as an active member of the ECU, succeeded in getting the wording changed to include others 'properly qualified'.

A Council for Chiropractic Education in Europe is

currently being formed, along the lines of the American CCE, with which any college of chiropractic will have to be registered before it can be recognized. (This will result in another curious anomaly: since the Council will be recognized by the similar councils already in existence, the Anglo-European College of Chiropractic, based in England, will be recognized by the American, Canadian, South African and Australian governments, but not by the British!)

Among the ECU member countries, Switzerland is the only one in which chiropractic is fully legislated; though legislation differs in the twenty-three cantons, six major insurance companies provide for 90 per cent recovery of fees. In West Germany chiropractic is governed by the law for *Heilpraktikern* ('health practitioners') which applies to other natural therapies, and federal reimbursement is available. In Italy there is government acknowledgement of chiropractic and federal reimbursement, provided treatment is carried out under the supervision of medical doctors. The few chiropractors in Spain have not achieved government recognition.

Chiropractic is legal under common law in Britain, Norway, Sweden, Denmark and the Netherlands; but there is government recognition in Norway and Denmark in so far as the state provides partial reimbursement of fees. Although the numbers are small (twenty-one chiropractors in 1983), Holland – a nation particularly open-minded in its views on alternatives – is rapidly moving towards acquiring government recognition, supported by the 9,000 members of its patients' association.

A Hellenic Chiropractors Association was formed with seven members in 1980. In 1986 a Spanish Chiropractors Association was formed with five members, and Finland, with nine members, became a full member of the ECU, while Cyprus, with four members, had applied to the ECU for membership.

France and Belgium come under Roman–Dutch law, under which chiropractic is technically illegal and chiropractors are banned from using X-rays (as is also the case in Sweden); French chiropractors have no trouble in getting X-rays taken by radiologists, who are privately organized. In France, indeed, there exists a curious situation, with more chiropractors in practice than in any other European country, and a school recently established in Paris. With typical French individuality, 130 qualified chiropractors belong to the French Chiropractors Association, while some 200 have chosen not to join.

Britain

225 chiropractors registered with the BCA, ninety-four with the Institute of Pure Chiropractic (1986). It is a far cry from the huckstering of the early USA chiropractors to the respectability projected today by the BCA and the Institute of Pure Chiropractic (IPC), with their well-run clinics and group practices, their ethical codes and disciplinary committees.

All of this might surprise the average member of the British public, many of whom believe that 'chiropractor' is American for osteopath, and some that chiropractors specialize in foot care! If chiropractic is relatively little known in Britain, this is largely owing to the historical accident that brought more osteopaths to England early in the century.

In 1925 nineteen chiropractors formed what was then the British Chiropractors (now Chiropractic) Association, which played a part in the formation of the ECU. In 1935 the ECU's 'official list' numbered 108 chiropractors in England, eighteen in Scotland and Wales, and eleven in Ireland.

Probably because of its small numbers, chiropractic in Britain has not suffered the same medical opposition as elsewhere. As in America, however, there have at times been disputes within the profession itself about principles and methods. (B. J. Palmer's 'Hole In One' caused controversy in England as well as in America.) European chiropractors, too, were divided between 'straights', who believed in practising chiropractic alone, and 'mixers', who wanted to use additional healing methods like homoeopathy and naturopathy, as well as mechanical devices; the British tended to favour the 'straights'.

There was also concern about training standards: in the early days chiropractors often learned their trade through apprenticeship to a practising chiropractor, or even by correspondence. In 1935 the ECU was deploring the existence of a British Chiropractic College in Barnes which offered a course of fifty-two extension or correspondence lessons.

After the Second World War, BCA membership had fallen from eighty to under forty. Since then, however, it has been growing slowly but steadily, and membership of the profession has been boosted over the last twenty years by the existence of the Anglo-European College of Chiropractic (AECC) in Bournemouth, formed in 1965 by some British chiropractors as a registered charity. After some initial lack of support from Europe the college turned to the ECU for assistance when it ran into financial difficulties, and since 1979 it has been truly European. One member of each of the ECU's national associations sits on its board of governors, and the Dean, Dr Arne Christensen, former president of the Danish Chiropractors Association, is also president of the ECU.

The AECC is enjoying steady growth: starting with twenty-five students, it currently has some 300 and aims at an intake of 400. Its full-time, four-year course is designed, according to the prospectus, 'to produce a primary contact practitioner with a sound integrated preclinical and clinical knowledge base, a high level of diagnostic and manual therapeutic skills, and an enthusiastic professional attitude

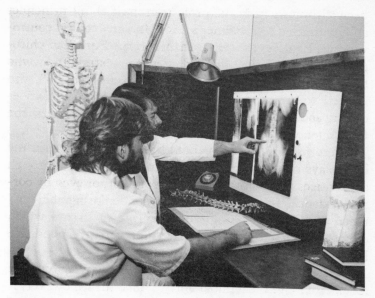

Studying the spine at the Anglo-European College of Chiropractic

towards chiropractic'. The curriculum, too long to quote in full, includes anatomy, physiology, biochemistry and radiography, as well as chiropractic techniques, and an optional recommended one- to two-year internship is being made compulsory. The establishment of the AECC has meant that Europeans no longer have to train in America or Canada. It attracts students from all over the world; around twenty-two nationalities were studying there in 1986.* It has seventy-six full- and part-time staff, including six doctors of medicine working as assistant lecturers and three as external examiners. A good relationship exists between the college and Poole General Hospital, whose consultant radiologist lectures to the students.

The 'enthusiasm' mentioned in the prospectus can be

*Fees in 1986 were around £2,800 a year. Some 76 per cent of British students get discretionary grants for their college fees from local education authorities. Danes and Norwegians are given mandatory grants by their governments.

detected among both graduates and students. The majority of students have benefited from chiropractic themselves or witnessed its benefits on friends or family. (One recent graduate is sorry that advertising is discouraged; he wants everyone to know what a good thing chiropractic is!) There is quite a high proportion (around 20 to 25 per cent) of mature students – a New Zealander recently graduated at the age of sixty-four, after a career as an engineer. Until recently there has been a heavy weighting of male students owing to an erroneous image of chiropractic as a heavy-duty form of manipulation requiring physical strength. This is on the turn; in 1986 the college had its highest-ever intake of women, totalling 41 per cent of new students.

During their final year students treat patients under close supervision (one tutor to four students) in the college clinic. In its sixteen treatment rooms, some 600 to 700 out-patients are treated every week for a reduced fee by experi-enced chiropractors as well as by students; three medical doctors assist in the diagnosis of problem cases. The college has a strongly scientific orientation; all students have to write a thesis on an aspect of research, and the AECC is currently (1986) trying to obtain acceptance of its training as a degree course.

There is a second school in Britain, quite distinct from the AECC. The McTimoney Chiropractic School (MCS) in Oxford was founded in 1972 and offers a four-year part-time course, along Open University lines; its professional body is the Institute of Pure Chiropractic. Its history and approach, which are very different from those of the AECC and the BCA, will be described fully in Part II, chapter 3. It has developed from very small beginnings, and seems set fair for further growth.

Despite its small numbers, chiropractic has a devoted following among those it has helped – usually after they have been through the medical mill without success. The clientele of both the BCA and the IPC includes some

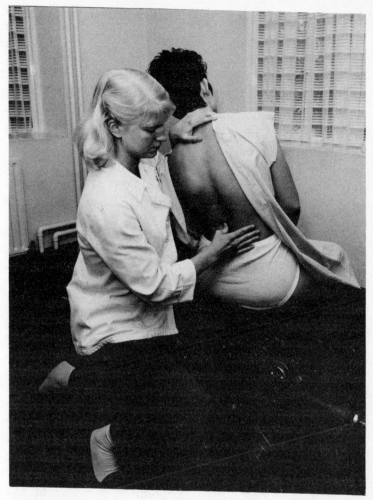

An increasing number of women are becoming chiropractors

well-known names in sport, politics and show-business, and even a few members of the medical profession. Doctors and surgeons who have experienced the results of chiropractic in themselves or their patients are referring an increasing number of patients to chiropractors. And the

therapy is being taken sufficiently seriously for the BCA to
be currently participating in a research programme authorized by the Medical Research Council to compare orthodox
and unorthodox medicine in the treatment of bad backs.

PART TWO

CHIROPRACTIC IN BRITAIN TODAY

CHAPTER ONE

THE BRITISH

CHIROPRACTIC ASSOCIATION

The British Chiropractic Association became a company limited by guarantee in 1984, when its name was changed. Set up to regulate the activities of its members and to promote the practice of chiropractic by qualified practitioners, its members believe firmly in the value of their therapy and want to make it more widely available. A related voluntary organization, the Chiropractic Advancement Association, formed in 1965 by people who have benefited from chiropractic, also aims to spread knowledge about the treatment and obtain its acceptance within the National Health Service. In 1975 the BCA applied for inclusion in the Professions Supplementary to Medicine, but this request was rejected with no reasons given. The BCA remains steadfast in its wish to obtain government recognition; meanwhile it is represented on the council of the Back Pain Association founded in 1968 to finance research into cures, causes and effects of back pain.

Although since the foundation of the Anglo-European College of Chiropractic British students have been able to study in England, many BCA members have graduated from colleges in the USA and Canada.

Chiropractic Theory and Practice

The BCA defines chiropractic as 'that independent branch

of medicine which specializes in mechanical disorders of the joints, particularly those of the spine, and their effects on the nervous system'.

The purpose of most chiropractic treatment is to treat subluxations, mainly in the spine, using appropriate techniques of adjustment. There can be some confusion about the word 'subluxation'; in medicine it specifically means a minor dislocation, but some chiropractors use it as an umbrella term to signify that there is something wrong with a joint (as osteopaths talk about 'lesions').

BCA chiropractors do not refer to 'displaced vertebrae', as Palmer did. '"Displacement" conjures up pictures of bones wildly out of place which need to be wrenched back into position,' a chiropractor explains. 'Chiropractic is much more subtle than that.' Basically, a subluxation occurs when, rather than being displaced, the facet joints which link the vertebrae become locked; this restricts movement and causes pain by irritating the nerves leading from the spinal cord to other parts of the body. 'We are not moving joints about; the changes that we make don't always show on X-rays – though we know we have made a change, and so does the patient. What we are doing is restoring mobility to the joints and improving their function.'

The word 'function' has also led to misunderstandings with doctors, who often refer to a 'functional' pain when they can discover nothing wrong with the patient (who is therefore labelled a hypochondriac!). Chiropractors use it to mean that there is something wrong with the mechanical function of the spine, 'as if an area of the spine has become jammed, like a locked drawer, which we loosen up'. These days chiropractors and pro-chiropractic doctors recognize that they may be speaking a different language and take this into account in their communications with one another.

In Britain, chiropractors have come to be regarded as back specialists. But according to George Walker, a former BCA president, 'Although the public primarily consult us for back pain, chiropractors are engineers who are dealing with the whole body machine.' Adjusting the spine directly affects the nervous system, increasing what chiropractors refer to as 'nerve supply': that is, they improve the nerves' efficiency to pass messages from the brain to the whole of the body. This, it is believed, can have a beneficial effect on over-all health; and because the central nervous system is linked with various organs via the peripheral and autonomic nervous systems, certain organic or visceral conditions, like headaches, digestive problems and asthma often respond well to adjustment. But although some American chiropractors still issue challenging statements along the lines of Palmer's '95 per cent of diseases are caused by subluxations', these are unlikely to be echoed in the UK. While some organic conditions can respond surprisingly well, cures are far from predictable, often occurring during treatment for another, more obvious problem. (These will be described in more detail in Part III, chapter 4.)

Chiropractic and Osteopathy

A question that is often asked is: 'How does chiropractic differ from osteopathy?' Although the two disciplines have developed in isolation from each other, both chiropractors and osteopaths tell me that more differences may be found between individual practitioners than between the two groups as a whole. Osteopaths treat the spine and nervous system for a range of problems similar to those that confront chiropractors. Theoretically there are technical differences: osteopaths are said to make more use of leverage; for example, they may release a locked joint in the middle or lower section of the spine by twisting the body and exerting pressure on the shoulders and hips. Chiropractors, by contrast, traditionally use a 'high-velocity low-amplitude thrust': that is, a short, sharp push on the joint itself. They believe that in general their adjustments are more 'specific', more precisely directed, than those carried out by osteopaths. But these days the distinctions are blurred, and similar techniques are used by both. As to the comparative effectiveness of the two, obviously some individuals are more gifted as manipulators than others but no trials have been undertaken to compare the two therapies. There are, however, likely to be wider variations in the skills and training of osteopaths, since there are a number of osteopathic schools, both full- and part-time; the word 'osteopath' can therefore signify both someone who has learned the technique at a weekend course and someone who has taken a full-time training.★

Given equal standards of training, the chief difference appears to be in the chiropractor's much more frequent use of X-rays in diagnosis.

Diagnosis and the Use of X-rays

A diagnostic session by a BCA chiropractor or by an osteopath with an equivalent training covers substantially the same ground, including case-history taking and physical, orthopaedic and neurological tests. Both are trained in making a differential diagnosis: that is, taking into account all possible causes of symptoms, not only musculo-skeletal problems. However, although qualified to read X-rays, osteopaths do not take them themselves, and will only have them taken by radiologists if they judge it absolutely neces-

★The General Council and Register of Osteopaths includes on its register around 800 osteopaths who have graduated from a full-time, four-year training at the British School of Osteopathy or the European School of Osteopathy, and medical doctors who have taken the thirteen-month postgraduate course at the London College of Osteopathic Medicine. Another reputable school is the British School of Naturopathy and Osteopathy, with around 280 osteopaths on its register.

sary. For BCA chiropractors, by contrast, X-rays are an important diagnostic aid. Eighty per cent have their own X-ray equipment, and they almost invariably take an X-ray on the patient's first visit in order to complete their diagnostic picture. There are three main reasons for this.

Firstly, and very importantly in their view, X-rays show up conditions for which manipulation is inappropriate. Secondly, X-rays help them to decide exactly where adjustments need to be made, and indicate the direction and force required. This, they say, enables them to carry out adjustments with a high degree of speed and accuracy. 'Some patients need a certain combination of adjustments to get them right,' says a chiropractor, 'and not all osteopaths meet these requirements.'

Thirdly, and no less importantly, X-rays enable chiropractors to detect the presence of conditions requiring medical treatment. There has been more than one instance of chiropractors correctly diagnosing problems that have been missed by other manipulators and even doctors. George Walker tells me of a patient who arrived walking on a fractured femur which had been missed by his GP and a hospital consultant! Sometimes a condition such as an early, undiagnosed tumour may be detected, in which case the chiropractor will immediately refer the patient to a doctor or consultant. They also find themselves correcting medical misdiagnoses. Chiropractor James Rousseau told me of one of his patients, a woman in her early forties, who had been on heavy pain-killers for fifteen years for what her doctor had diagnosed as osteoarthritis of the hip. On X-raying his patient – which her doctor had not done – he found that there was no osteoarthritis in the joint, but that she had serious mechanical problems in the pelvis and lower back, which could be treated by adjustment. (Although this was a slow process, she was able to give up her pain-killers soon after beginning treatment.)

Osteopaths are concerned about the effects of irradiation

from X-rays, and hold that other symptoms, such as tissue changes, should alert manipulators to the presence of conditions they are not qualified to treat. (McTimoney chiropractors also hold this view.) BCA chiropractors are convinced that taking a minimal number of X-rays is justified in the interests of the patient's health. Although it is probably fairly rare for serious conditions to remain undiagnosed when patients visit 'alternative' therapists, it has been known to happen. The results can be tragic for the patient, and also arm the medical establishment with a stick with which to belabour the alternatives – even though, unfortunately, both GPs and hospital doctors are not perfect in this respect. (A pro-chiropractic surgeon says: 'The number of things that ordinary doctors miss is alarming and amazing.')

Chiropractors are determined not to miss anything. It has been suggested that in the litigation-conscious USA chiropractors take more X-rays than they need to, as insurance against lawsuits. (They are also obliged to take them by Medicare, the American health insurance scheme.) British chiropractors do try to keep them to a minimum. They are obviously well aware of the dangers of irradiation and make every effort to avoid taking X-rays that could affect those people and parts of the body at particular risk – that is, children and adolescents, foetuses, the eyes, and the reproductive organs in adults of child-producing age. (If the pelvis has to be X-rayed, these organs can be protected by gonad shields.)

In addition to X-rays, BCA chiropractors are qualified if necessary to read CT-scans, take blood and urine tests and blood-pressure readings, and to read the physical signs (skin quality, breath odour, etc.) that could indicate faulty nutrition or digestive problems. They may not always carry out chemical tests themselves; many patients will have been through them already, and it is often simpler to refer a patient to a hospital for tests requiring a lot of time and equipment. But their understanding of the significance of the results helps them to come to an accurate diagnosis.

Thus chiropractors obtain a very complete diagnostic picture – more complete, they believe, than some medical diagnoses as far as the spine and joints are concerned. Many GPs do not physically examine the spine, and if a patient is sent to see a specialist, the latter may be over-specialized. 'The trouble with medicine at the moment is that it's fragmented,' says a chiropractor. 'The orthopaedic surgeon is interested in the pathology of the bone, and the neurologist in the pathology of the nerve. And there's a grey area where a bone or joint is irritating a nerve, which is not covered by either. That loophole is what chiropractic covers; we are specialists in analysing how the machinery is irritating a nerve.'

Variations on a Theme

Probably no two chiropractors treat patients identically; as with any group of human beings, their particular abilities, interests and personal charm is likely to vary. Some are pure body mechanics; some take a deep personal interest in their patients' over-all welfare. Some develop particular gifts and become specialists in specific areas such as sports injuries or the treatment of children, or acquire a reputation for being 'good' with problems like migraine. Their techniques vary, too; their training arms them with a wide range from which to choose, and individual chiropractors have their own favourites which work best for them.

The main technique is adjustment, in which the chiropractor places his hands on or near the appropriate joint, and applies a small amount of force in order to restore its function and mobility. Another commonly used technique is traction, which involves using manual techniques to stretch the spine. Other techniques are used as and when appropriate, including soft-tissue techniques, similar to

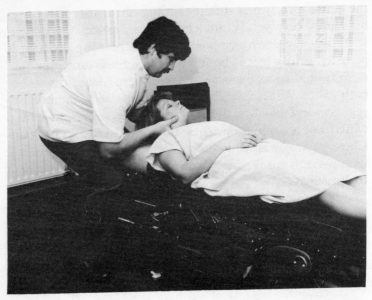

Treating a patient in the Anglo-European College of Chiropractic clinic

gentle massage, which are used to release tight ligaments or muscles in spasm. Tender spots, called 'trigger points', can be found within the muscles, where the chiropractor can sense clear changes in the muscle texture; these often correspond with acupuncture points. Research has shown that when muscles are in spasm their chemical constituents are changed at these points; by stimulating them the circulation of the blood and the lymphatic system are stimulated, helping to clear out toxins and relaxing the whole muscle.

Some chiropractors simply practise what they have learned in college; others take postgraduate courses to acquire further techniques. One which seems to be enjoying a current vogue is the sacro-occipital technique, which focuses on the nerve connections between the head and the bottom of the spine. The theory is similar to that of an osteopathic technique called cranial osteopathy, although the actual practice is different; the cranial osteopath uses his hands very gently, the chiropractor places the patient with the pelvis lying on wedge-shaped blocks, so that it is adjusted gently by the body's own weight. Both techniques stem from the same source, the work of an American osteopath called William Sutherland, and both are intended to regulate and balance the flow of the cerebro-spinal fluid which bathes and nourishes the spinal cord and brain. Chiropractors trained in the sacro-occipital technique use it with patients for whom it is appropriate at certain stages of treatment.

Applied Kinesiology

Another popular and fairly recent development, also taught at postgraduate courses in Britain, is Applied Kinesiology (AK). This is chiefly a system of diagnosis, developed by Dr George Goodheart, an American chiropractor. He says that his discovery came about by 'serendipity', though it seems to have evolved from his acute sense of observation. He claims that there are very few true cases of spontaneous muscle spasm; that where a muscle is in spasm the muscle on the opposite side of the body will be weak, and that the reasons for this weakness may be nutritional or psychological as well as structural. True health depends on an equally balanced triad of structure, chemistry and mentality; when a chiropractic adjustment does not 'hold', there is likely to be an imbalance in the person's nutrition or psychology, or a pathological degeneration of the 'motor unit' (that is, the vertebra, disc, adjacent vertebra and attachments).

Dr Goodheart found that different muscles relate to specific organs and bodily systems; by testing their strength a chiropractor can not only tell whether a person's problem is structural, nutritional or emotional, but whether it relates to the lymphatic, circulatory, nervous or glandular systems, or even to a blockage in the acupuncture meridians. (Dr Goodheart has found that every meridian has an associated point on the spine.) This indicates the type of treatment required. It is a very accurate form of diagnosis, says Dr Goodheart, since 'the body cannot lie' – that is, its reactions to specific tests indicate exactly what is wrong, and where. There are also some specific AK techniques for balancing the two sides of the body and brain (it is said to be helpful for dyslexia), and even for treating emotional trauma.

A number of alternative therapists today use AK, or a simplified version of it, 'Touch for Health'. This was developed by a colleague of Dr Goodheart's, John Thie, with the object of providing a basic form of AK which could be practised by lay people on their friends and family. Dr Goodheart supported this at one time, but 'found the teaching produced such enthusiasm that people started to practise it other than with their families' and separated himself from it. In England the Touch for Health organization stresses that it is a health support system for lay people, not a complete system of health care. About a third of those who have taken its weekend courses are already practising medicine or alternative therapies and find it useful, for example, for testing dietary and vitamin requirements; some have gone on to take the much lengthier AK training. In New Zealand, Touch for Health has become very popular with doctors.

Many of Dr Goodheart's findings have been substantiated by research (although not all of this is considered reliable), and a number of British chiropractors have taken courses in AK, using it as a diagnostic aid in deciding on appropriate treatment or for testing food and vitamin requirements. The latter is done by placing a sample of the food or a pill in the patient's mouth and testing the appropriate muscles; if the product is 'bad' for the patient the muscle will weaken. Some chiropractors are cautious about placing total reliance on this, however, feeling that the results may be affected by their own or the patient's preconceptions about their dietary needs.

It is a fascinating subject, too complex to go into fully here.* It will be interesting to see whether it continues to expand in Britain as it has in the USA, where some 80 to 90 per cent of chiropractors use it, as well as medical doctors, dentists, and so on.

Beyond the BCA

An American chiropractor, Dr Milo Siewert, was present in the mid 1960s when Dr Goodheart began lecturing on AK. 'At the time we thought he'd lost his marbles, it seemed really kooky! Then a few of us started using it, and gosh, it did work!' Dr Siewert, a kindly, gentle person who is also a qualified medical doctor, now runs the Bournemouth Centre for Complementary Medicine which offers residential holistic treatment for people with all kinds of problems, including – somewhat controversially – some cancer patients. Dr Siewert stresses the importance of nutrition. 'If there is a nerve interference, particularly in the spinal column, then nutrition or medication will not correct it until you set that nerve free and enable that body to function correctly. If it's not from that source, but maybe from malnutrition or nutrition not compatible for this particular person, then all the adjustments in the world are not going to straighten this person out. As chiropractic evolved we found that, by prescribing vitamins and minerals, adjustments were holding better, there was a longer period between adjustments, and patients were feeling better all round.' At the Bournemouth Centre,

*For further information, see *Applied Kinesiology* by Tom and Carole Valentine, Thorson's Publishers, Wellingborough and New York, 1985.

chiropractic and AK are just two of a whole range of alternative therapies on offer, including physical therapies, meditation, yoga and hypnotherapy.

Another American-trained chiropractor, David Tansley, treats patients chiropractically but also, if appropriate, uses homoeopathy, Bach Flower Remedies, and radionics. Radionics is a system of healing and diagnosis involving specially designed instruments which may be used in the patient's absence, using a bloodspot or lock of hair as a link. Among other uses, it is said to be able to identify the causes of disease, and to determine the state of the body's invisible energy system, or *chakras*. At one time it was used by many American chiropractors and taught in some colleges. However, by the time David Tansley went to a chiropractic college in Los Angeles in the early 1950s, the teaching had become much more mechanistic and radionics had been made illegal, largely because it was scientifically inexplicable. 'Something that deals with electro-magnetic fields is OK by the establishment,' Mr Tansley comments, 'but when you start dealing with the life force, which is not the same thing, you get jumped on.' In this country radionics is not 'jumped on' (despite efforts to do so earlier in the century); nor is treating the life force through another 'non-scientific' means, such as hand healing.

Even in America, the tide is turning; one American chiropractor believed, before he was treated by one, that all chiropractors were 'quacks'. Since his training at Palmer College, he has developed his own techniques to the point where he treats the spine by adjusting the energy field outside the physical body. He says that he can get extremely good results without touching the body at all, though 'because this blows most people's concept of reality' he usually makes physical adjustments after treating the energy field.

You are unlikely to meet with such unconventional methods among BCA chiropractors. The BCA disci-

plined one of its members who was using a pendulum and a
lock of the patient's hair for diagnosis, and another who was
practising spiritual healing. The objection was not to the
practices in themselves; the BCA recognizes that many
people make a contribution to health, but holds to the view
that someone who goes to a chiropractor should expect and
be given chiropractic treatment.

Healing the Body . . .

One of the attractions of alternative and complementary
medicine is holism, the philosophy of treating the patient as
a whole being, not as a collection of separate parts each
requiring the attention of a different specialist. It also em-
braces the concept of the patient not only as body but as
mind and spirit, within a particular environment, whose
well-being also depends on his participation in his own
healing process. How far chiropractic fulfils this definition
depends on both the practitioner and the problem being
treated – after all, someone with tennis elbow is more interested in pain relief than soul-searching.

As far as serious musculo-skeletal problems are concerned, chiropractic certainly shares with other alternative
or complementary therapies the principle that the path to
healing lies in treating causes, not symptoms, and that this
necessitates looking at the whole person. First, chiropractors will usually examine the patient's entire musculo-
skeletal system, not just the area that hurts. Even taken as a
machine, all our body parts interrelate; neck problems are
often connected with pelvic problems, for instance, and bad
posture can affect the whole spine. Most BCA chiropractors will given commonsense advice about diet, without
going as far as advocating fasting and raw food; some, however, have a particular interest in nutrition, and give
detailed guidance when appropriate. Others have gone on

to take additional training in subjects such as counselling, acupuncture, herbalism or homoeopathy, and may offer patients a choice or combination of treatments.

By and large, the majority tread a relatively narrow path, preferring excellence in one area to an over-diversification of resources. Steve Carpenter, for example, is a chiropractor who clearly cares about his patients and supports the concept of holism, but who at the same time believes that the therapist should not try to be a jack-of-all-trades. He is, he says, 'a firm believer that chiropractors should be treating primarily mechanical musculo-skeletal disorders. You generally find that if the nervous system is working properly you can begin to get rid of a lot of psychological stress and to cope with nutritional problems as well, simply because the nerves are working that much more efficiently. If it's going to speed up the body's response I would give some psychological and nutritional advice. But if it becomes obvious that the patient's *primary* problem is chemical (nutritional or otherwise), or psychological, I refer them to a specialist, such as a naturopath or herbalist, or for counselling.'

At the same time, most chiropractors would like to be recognized as more than 'back doctors'. South African James Rousseau trained at the AECC after a career as a karate instructor (which he still continues); he points out that health is not just taking care of pain. 'If you start getting good results fixing knees, you get a reputation as a good knee-fixer and you'll get a lot of patients with bad knees! It's a great pity. I prefer to work on the level of health rather than on the level of disease, not just curing pain as crisis therapy. Health is an on-going thing; it means operating at optimum functioning. One very important part is that patients have to accept responsibility for their health; all I can do is help them. So if they have a problem in the pelvic area I do the adjustments that create the right environment for the healing to take place; but patients must be aware that if there is a weakness in the back they really have to take care of that, and not go and lounge about in bad chairs. I think the future role of a chiropractor must be in patient management, counselling and preventative care.'

... Mind ...

Another attraction for patients that chiropractic shares with other alternatives is the amount of time and attention the therapist is able to give to patients, in contrast with the average six minutes per consultation the GP is able to allot. This in itself can be healing for people with long-standing pain, who may already have struggled slowly through the hospital system with little benefit. Some people express enormous relief when their pain is taken seriously, when they are no longer told they 'have to live with it'; relief in itself can help tense muscles to relax.

Even if chiropractors restrict themselves to mechanical disorders, this does not mean that the patient is treated like a machine. A good chiropractor is good at dealing with people, and aware of the importance of his relationship with his patients. (Steve Carpenter says that his AECC training made him better able to communicate with people; conversely, some students drop out when they realize what dealing with people all day really involves!) Established chiropractors often take on something of the role of the traditional family GP.

A good chiropractor is a good communicator and a good listener. He needs to be able to explain to patients, who may range from manual workers to orthopaedic surgeons, what he is doing to them and why. In addition, for accurate diagnosis he must ask the right questions – and *hear* the answers. Questioning patients may require a degree of empathy and intuition: people whose pain has not been satisfactorily accounted for by their doctors may hesitate to ask what they really want to know. George Walker sometimes finds himself asking patients: 'What do *you* think is wrong with you?' They may be disconcerted by the question, he says, since it's one they're not used to. 'But I often find people are afraid that they have cancer, or a heart disease, or a thrombosis. Setting someone at ease and convincing them that is not the case enables their anxiety to settle.' He adds: 'When I first started practice I wouldn't have asked that question, because I had a mechanistic approach. I was constantly dealing with patients who had been told they were neurotic because the doctor couldn't account for their pain; I treated them physically and they got well. But now I realize that by getting rid of the patient's pain you create an enormously powerful relationship which allows them to shift their burden of anxiety. The stress-related elements are therefore subdued, and the patient starts to recover.'

In some cases people may suffer from emotional problems severe enough to impede their recovery. A woman returning from treatment to a difficult domestic situation, for example, may automatically tense up and undo the chiropractor's work. If this situation has not emerged at the diagnostic session the chiropractor may need to reassess his first diagnosis to find out why she is not responding as she should. Some chiropractors have trained as counsellors; others prefer to continue to treat the patient's body, while suggesting that they should seek professional help for their emotions, either referring them direct or suggesting that they ask their GP to refer them to someone suitable.

Often just listening is enough. A woman chiropractor finds that some of her patients begin to unburden their problems as soon as they lie down on her table. 'I just listen,' she says. 'I don't give advice unless they ask for it. I think they talk to me because I don't know them and they can tell me what they wouldn't tell their best friend. I used to take my patients' problems home with me, but when I got married I had to leave them at work. As long as I'm with them I give them the best that I can.'

... and Spirit?

How far do BCA chiropractors incorporate the 'spirit' into their treatment? According to Palmer's original concept there is a cyclical relationship between Universal and Innate Intelligence mediated via the nervous system; the harmonious function of this cycle is health, and any inter-ruption in the relationship leads to dis-ease. This philoso-phy is taught in the first year at the AECC, but not as dogma, and among BCA members can be found a com-plete range of philosophies, from the totally scientific to the totally spiritual.

As with medicine, the chiropractic profession has become increasingly knowledgeable about the actual mechanisms of pain and the nervous system; as George Walker puts it: 'Dwelling on the philosophy has become less important, because the philosophy is no longer a juggernaut riding on the back of a small vehicle called science; science has grown and the philosophy has diminished.'

Hence some chiropractors dismiss the concept of Innate Intelligence as 'inane rubbish', or simply of no value. 'Some people have the feeling that in order to justify what we do we have to invoke some sort of spiritualistic concept,' says a chiropractor who entered the profession after becom-ing disillusioned with a training in radionics, hand healing and colour therapy. 'There are very rational, tangible argu-ments for what we do. The reason I am still a chiropractor is because it works.'

I would have thought that 'Innate Intelligence' is simply nineteenth-century terminology for the life force, the body's own self-healing ability which is recognized in all natural therapies; and probably many chiropractors would agree with this. I also see no reason why a Universal Intelligence should not operate through chiropractors, doctors or scientists. The woman chiropractor quoted above favours the scientific viewpoint; but at times, she says, with some patients, and particularly when she is using soft-tissue techniques, 'I feel very calm and I do wonder if I am also doing healing.'

Steve Carpenter believes that the philosophy is important to chiropractic, and should be given its due. 'The reason chiropractors are so strong worldwide in the field of alternative medicine is because of their philosophy, the fact that we are humble enough to know that when we make a correction to a body, no matter how artistic or skilful it may be ... it is not only the skill of the chiropractor that is getting the patient better. We are opening the channels for the spiritual aspects of the body to heal and harmonize with the environment.' He believes that the strength of chiropractic lies in its combination of a spiritual approach *and* a scientific basis.

Whatever their beliefs, chiropractors are unlikely to preach them at their patients. My own impression is that there is a widespread spiritual hunger today, and that for many who patronize alternative therapies the spiritual aspect is one of the attractions. Whether spoken of or not, when a therapist's work is underpinned by a spiritual philosophy this is liable to convey itself to patients, and I cannot see why this should conflict with scientific facts. George Walker is able to encompass both. 'As a scientist,' he says, 'because I cannot measure some things, I am not able to consider that they therefore don't exist. And as a practising Christian I don't have any difficulty with the philosophy, which is very akin to Christianity. It doesn't dominate my clinical thinking, but it certainly pervades my personality and relationship with patients.'

CHAPTER TWO

THE McTIMONEY

CHIROPRACTIC SCHOOL

If chiropractic is an alternative therapy, the McTimoney Chiropractic School (MCS) could be described as the alternative to the alternative. It descended from Palmer's teachings along a separate branch-line from the main American and European organizations, and its aims, teaching and techniques differ from those of the British Chiropractic Association (BCA) and the Anglo-European College of Chiropractic (AECC). The AECC in Bournemouth, with its four-year full-time course, aims to produce 'primary health care practitioners' – chiropractors to whom patients can refer themselves direct and be given a thorough clinical diagnosis, including X-rays. The part-time course provided by the MCS produces chiropractors who prefer to work as independent specialists in a complementary or supplementary role to medical doctors. Both schools train their students in skilled palpation and manipulation, based on sound mechanical principles; but where the AECC emphasizes science, the MCS also encourages intuition and spiritual values; where the AECC trains students in a variety of techniques, MCS practitioners concentrate mainly on one. Chiropractic is an art and a science. 'We are craftsmen, not academics,' says one of their recent graduates. Judging by the approval of most of their patients, as craftsmen they are skilled, effective and caring.

John McTimoney and the Founding of the School

John McTimoney was yet another eccentric character in

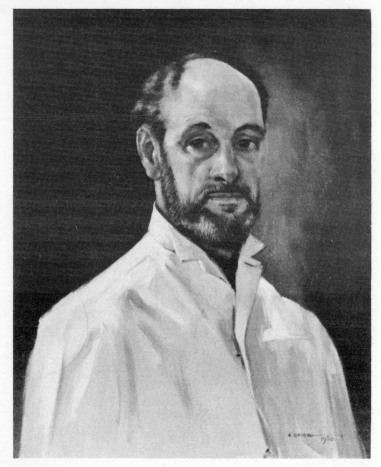

John McTimoney, founder of the Oxfordshire College of Chiropractic

the history of chiropractic: gifted, creative, generous, unbusinesslike, and a rebel against authority. He left a legacy of a gentle, holistic method of manipulation whose practitioners are steadily growing in both numbers and medical approval.

In 1939, as a young man, McTimoney was working on a farm when a fall from a ladder forced him to give up heavy work. In 1940 he joined the Air Ministry as a technical artist, for which he was already qualified. (He had also previously trained as a silversmith.) In 1942 he began losing the use of his arms as a result of the earlier fall; the only medical treatment offered was an operation, with poor prospects of recovery. Some years earlier his wife had been cured of catarrhal deafness by a Mr Ashford of Birmingham, a BCA chiropractor who had trained under D. D. Palmer; McTimoney went to him for treatment and was also cured. During his talks with Mr Ashford he became fascinated by chiropractic; he was struck by the logic of its philosophy of cause and effect and became eager to learn it himself. At that time the BCA was composed entirely of graduates from the Palmer College, Davenport, who were forbidden to teach in the UK; anyone wanting to train had to go to Iowa – which McTimoney could not afford.

In 1944 John McTimoney was working in Oxford for the Ministry of Works; the local chiropractor recommended by Mr Ashford was Dr Mary Walker (Doctor of Chiropractic), a former medical nursing matron who had trained at Palmer College under B. J. Palmer; despite the Palmer College ruling, she planned to start a school of chiropractic in Oxford on her return to Britain in 1936 – she was a determined lady. As a former matron she sought the approval of her local doctors, but its failure to materialize, together with the onset of the Second World War, put the matter into abeyance.

The ageing Dr Walker was none the less anxious to pass on her skills. She had started training one student in 1947 – Joan Nind, who was still in part-time practice in Oxford in 1986. John McTimoney had already relieved his wife, at a time when Dr Walker was unavailable, 'of a very acute attack of pain and temperature with the loss of use of her left arm ... by finding which vertebra was responsible for the disorder and copying what I had witnessed so many times [he had watched Dr Walker treating his family], adjusting the vertebrae successfully and relieving my wife to the extent that she was able to visit Dr Walker the next morning'.* Treating one's nearest and dearest without training is not a procedure to be generally recommended! However, Dr Walker recognized his keenness to learn and decided to teach him herself, with two Doctors of Chiropractic as his examiners. His training, which he describes as 'comprehensive and severe', followed the curriculum of Dr Walker's planned school and took nearly three years.

In 1951 McTimoney started what was soon a flourishing practice in Banbury, though it was not likely to make him rich since he often treated patients for nothing. Stories are told of him treating people at midnight, and then driving them home himself. He evolved and developed one chiropractic technique in particular; he also adapted it for the treatment of animals and developed a flourishing animal practice.†

He was so successful with both humans and animals that he was asked to take on students himself, which he seems to have done with open-heartedness and a total lack of concern for profit-making. In 1972, with the help of his wife and two daughters (both of whom now work as chiropractors), he opened the Oxfordshire School of Chiropractic with fourteen students. Regarding mature students with some experience of life as the best material, he created a part-time course enabling students to continue to work while studying. He assessed applicants on their personal qualities rather than their academic prowess; as a result, new students of whom 'Mac' approved were taken on in mid course, while those who could not pay were told: 'Pay me when you can!' In 1980, at the age of sixty-six, he died of a heart attack brought on by overwork. His widow did not wish to continue running the School, but a group of former students, including an experienced businessman,

*From an account written by John McTimoney in the late 1960s.
†John McTimoney's work with animals is described in Part I I I, chapter 7.

wanted to see his work continued. With Mrs McTimoney's agreement they took the School over for a nominal fee and reorganized it along more conventional lines. They renamed it the McTimoney Chiropractic School in his memory.

The MCS Training

The School has deliberately been kept small, with an intake limited to twenty-six part-time students a year. Academic qualifications, although desirable, are not essential for entrance, being regarded as less important than compassion and a dedication to healing people. These qualities are assessed by the staff who invite applicants to the School for the day, getting to know them in a relaxed atmosphere. Ninety per cent of the trainees are mature students (the average age is thirty-four) who have been through other careers, and, interestingly, the majority are women (70 per cent in 1986). A new intake of students may range from people with degrees in biology, people with nursing or medical qualifications or training in other alternative therapies, to people with no qualifications or experience of treating patients. Many are themselves grateful patients who are attracted by the School's atmosphere and philosophy – a BBC employee taking the course told me that joining the School was like 'coming home'. Most are in full-time jobs, and the drop-out rate of only 7 per cent over four years says much for their dedication.

Theoretical work includes lectures and tutorials at the School in basic physiology and anatomy, with guidelines to differential diagnosis, and as much home study in the form of reading matter and taped lectures as students working in their spare time can manage – probably a year-round average of fifteen hours a week. Twenty to thirty examinations

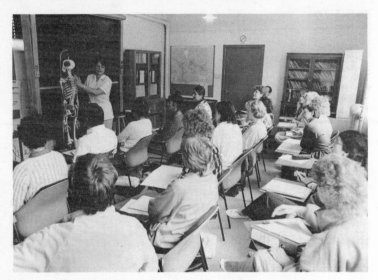

A lecture at the McTimoney Chiropractic School

and tests a year are conducted throughout the course on a progressive basis.

The practical training is the vital core of the course; students visit the School once a month to be trained in palpating and adjusting techniques, and to develop a high degree of manual and intuitive sensitivity. In addition to their days at the School, some students meet voluntarily to practise palpation and adjustment and to help each other study. For practical instruction the School provides one teacher to six students, reducing to one teacher to two students in the third year, and one teacher to each student in the clinical work during the advanced stage of the course. In the third and fourth years students work under supervision in the ten McTimoney Teaching Clinics around the country, where patients are treated for a reduced fee. At the end of the fourth year, after passing all their theoretical tests and examinations, the students face a stiff assessment of their clinical abilities; they are assessed not only on their tech-

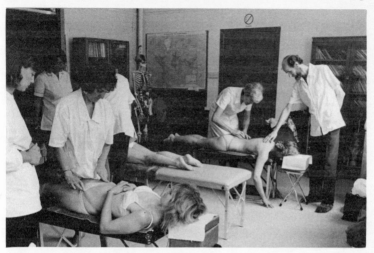

Practical instruction at the McTimoney Chiropractic School

nique but on their whole approach, including chiropractic explanations, record-taking, presentation, and manner with patients. (AECC students are assessed on similar aspects of care.) Successful graduates use the initials 'C.P.' (Chiropractic Practitioner). Carrying on the tradition started by John McTimoney, there is an optional further twelve months' training in animal manipulation, which may only be undertaken by MCS graduates.

The School was registered as a charity, the McTimoney Chiropractic School Trust, in 1986. The professional body of the School is the Institute of Pure Chiropractic (IPC) – 'pure' refers to the fact that practitioners use hands-only chiropractic, with no mechanical aids. It was set up to support qualified McTimoney chiropractors, and governs the code of ethics and standards of practice of its members; it offers associate and full membership (A.I.P.C. and, after three years of practice, M.I.P.C.). It is currently under the chairmanship of former professional cricketer Michael Mence, now Assistant Secretary to the MCC and ICC, an enthusiastic former patient. He was forced to give up cricket and 'learn to live with back pain' after medical tests, manipulation and four months in plaster had failed to cure what was diagnosed as 'disc lesions'. Some five or six years later he was put in touch with a McTimoney chiropractor who produced instant relief, and has continued to do so if ever Mence's back trouble recurs. As Chairman, his aim is to achieve national recognition for the MCS.

McTimoney Treatment and Its Results

IPC chiropractors examine the whole of the body at every session, holding that there is a vital connection between different parts of the body which should not therefore be treated in isolation from one another. In palpating a patient's spine, the chiropractor looks for misalignments in the vertebrae, which indicate subluxations requiring adjustment. While employing more than one technique to treat the whole body, they adjust vertebrae using the 'toggle recoil', a technique which originated with Palmer and was developed by John McTimoney. It consists of an extremely light and fast movement – a thrust, torque and recoil – of the hands on a specific part of the bone. It requires accuracy and expertise, and acquiring the necessary muscular control demands a lot of practice. Carried out correctly it is usually painless; performed incorrectly or slowly (as it sometimes is by non-qualified manipulators) it could be painful.

Bronwen Herbertson, one of the MCS lecturers, is a qualified physiotherapist as well as an IPC chiropractor with ten years' experience in full-time practice. She explains: 'What the treatment does in simple mechanical terms is to restore bones to their correct resting positions. Except with severe trauma, bones do not move from A to B, but in patients treated by this method the bones feel twisted away from their correct positions when the body is palpated at rest. When a patient is in agony it is usual for the spinous process* of a relevant vertebra, or several vertebrae, to feel, on palpation, to be half an inch away from the patient's midline.' Many misalignments are much more subtle, requiring a lot of sensitivity to detect, but they can still cause pain by compressing or stretching nerves, while adjustment relieves pain and restores the spine to normal functioning. 'In my experience,' says Mrs Herbertson, 'the severity of the distortions in the bony structure parallels the degree of disability in the patient. Correcting these distortions in the vast majority of cases restores the function of the nervous system to normal, and thereby the patient's health.'

As we have already seen, theories about what occurs during an adjustment have not been scientifically proven, but chiropractors and patients know what their own experience is. The toggle recoil technique is so light that, although the chiropractor knows he has brought about a change, patients sometimes wonder at the time whether anything is being done at all, and are surprised at its effects. The belief is that the body responds to 'gentle messages', and this certainly seems to be the case.

In 1983 IPC practitioners sent out 4,000 questionnaires to past and present patients asking for their assessment of their treatment and its results. The 3,000 completed forms that were returned make quite impressive reading. Most of these patients describe definite and measurable improvements in a wide range of musculo-skeletal disorders, and speak highly of the care and attention they have received from their chiropractors. In addition, many patients have been cured of unexpected problems, among which migraine and headaches are frequently mentioned.

*The spinous processes are the parts of the vertebrae which can be seen as slightly protuberant 'knobs' going down the spine.

Analysis, Not Diagnosis

The MCS's lack of insistence on academic qualifications and comparatively abbreviated diagnostic training have drawn some criticism from BCA chiropractors with their medically oriented training. But, as mentioned above, the MCS does not aim to produce practitioners who will replace doctors, and regards 'certain medical procedures as being the province of the medical profession'.

McTimoney practitioners don't claim to diagnose in the medical sense, using Palmer's word 'analysis' for their examination of the patient. They do not take X-rays; John McTimoney shared the view of many alternative therapists that X-rays can be damaging and are to be avoided.* The School emphasizes the development of manual sensitivity and dexterity, summed up in the statements: 'If you can't palpate it you can't adjust it', and 'X-rays are 2-D, fingers are 3-D'. X-rays, they say, do not necessarily show what they need to know in order to perform correct adjustments. There are instances, however, when IPC chiropractors are happy to see X-rays that have already been taken, or will even have them taken – particularly, for example, if someone has had a previous accident or operation. There have also been instances of IPC chiropractors correcting a medical diagnosis by touch alone, as in the case of a patient whose medically diagnosed 'multiple sclerosis' symptoms turned out to be caused by a subluxated vertebra in the neck causing pressure on the spinal cord, which the chiropractor was able to treat. The most common medical 'misdiagnosis', says one, is, 'You'll just have to live with your

*The arguments for and against X-rays could ping-pong back and forth forever. There are cases in which X-rays have shown conditions which could not be palpated, and others in which palpation has shown up conditions invisible on X-rays. One or two X-rays do not create high enough dosages of radiation to cause damage, except in the instances cited on page 44; at the same time it is preferable not to have them taken unnecessarily, as repeated radiation dosages can build up to a damaging level over time.

back-ache!', when in fact the patient's pain can be cured by adjustment.

Since they do not present themselves to the public as primary health care therapists, they prefer their patients to have had a medical diagnosis before coming to them; when possible, most like to work in cooperation with doctors. In fact the majority of their patients, disillusioned with or distrustful of conventional medicine, are self-referred; 99 per cent of them arrive with musculo-skeletal problems which have already been medically diagnosed, but not medically relieved. However, not all back and joint pains stem from the musculo-skeletal system; they may relate, for instance, to heart problems, diabetes, kidney or gall-bladder malfunction, or cancer of the bone. IPC chiropractors are alert to the possibility that some anti-doctor patient will turn up 'off the street' with a serious undiagnosed condition. They should be able to detect, from the patient's general health and other symptoms, whether a 'sinister' condition is present – some have indeed recognized such cases – and if in any doubt about the patient's diagnosis they refer them back to their doctor. (When I first visited an IPC chiropractor she pointed out a tiny but odd-looking mole on my leg which I was unaware of, and suggested that I should have it medically checked.)

Like BCA chiropractors, some IPC chiropractors have a special interest or training in subjects like nutrition, counselling and acupuncture, and some have taken Touch for Health courses; they will incorporate these methods into their treatment if the case requires it. Others will refer patients, where appropriate, to nutritionists, Applied Kinesiologists, counsellors, and so on.

Many are also trying, with some success, to build up communication with their local GPs – for example, by sending a report to the doctor of a new patient, whether medically referred or not. And doctors who are aware of the chiropractor's abilities do refer patients. After hearing many tales of unsympathetic medical men, it was refreshing to talk with Dr Mark Drury, a GP whose group practice refers suitable cases to IPC chiropractors, osteopaths or acupuncturists.

'I found out about it through patients who'd initially been spontaneously,' he told me, 'and after visiting the School once or twice I began to refer patients direct. We tend to be fairly selective about the people we refer, and normally take them through the conventional medical investigations, and often conventional treatment too, before raising the subject of alternative medicine; I would certainly be unhappy referring someone with back pain for primary treatment to a chiropractor without knowing there was no sinister lesion or tumour of the spine. But when we are faced with the alternative of having to ask the patient to wait three or four months in considerable pain for the orthopaedic surgeon to tell them to go away and rest, there's not much more we have at our disposal, and chiropractors certainly come up with results. The results are very good, and we have had no complaints at all. The approach and the time the chiropractor can spend with people is clearly of benefit, too; people feel generally better for seeing someone who will look at the whole person.'

A Holistic Philosophy

The concept of holism, that you cannot reduce man to the sum of his parts, is important to the teaching, which has a strong spiritual emphasis. The idea of Innate Intelligence seems more acceptable to MCS graduates than to some of the more scientifically oriented BCA chiropractors; whether one regards this as retrograde, or whether Palmer himself was ahead of his time, must be a matter of personal opinion. Certainly a spiritual and intuitive approach is in keeping with the mood of many members of the public in the 1980s, when spiritual healing, for instance, is undergoing an expansion of interest from both the public and the medical profession.

In philosophical terms the patient is seen as a spiritual as well as a physical and emotional being. 'Man is still a mystery,' says Stan Harding, one of the School's directors. 'You can look at all the tissues and organs and systems of the body in a laboratory; man is much more than that. Palmer wrote that you cannot treat the body without affecting the mind and spirit. My personal belief is that a change in human consciousness can be effected by chiropractic; things actually change at a very subtle level and suddenly people see things differently. There is a known esoteric relationship between the spine and spiritual awareness and growth. Some patients have said, "Since I've had the treatment I've been able to manage better with my life: my perception has changed." '

In the questionnaires returned by patients, a number report an increase in well-being and emotional calm, and even a feeling of euphoria following treatment. Whether these effects derive from the relief of pain, the attentiveness of the chiropractor, or are the result of the treatment on the nervous system – or the spirit – is probably not provable at this stage of medical and scientific knowledge.

As with BCA chiropractors, there are variations in the degree to which spiritual ideas are accepted – and a mutual tolerance of differing views. Bronwen Herbertson, who works closely with Stan Harding in running the School, has a more down-to-earth approach. She says: 'Whether we work directly on the spirit or not I have my doubts. But if you relieve physical discomfort you release the person to do what they want to do and open horizons they thought were shut to them; patients often claim they feel ten years younger. I think the McTimoney technique is the greatest curative and prophylactic healing treatment I have encountered in the twenty years I have been in health care.'

Among current students is a doctor, formerly a GP, who comments: 'If you are treating people with chiropractic you have to have a particular belief system about spinal manipulation and its effects upon the function of the body. For instance, "increasing nerve supply" is gobbledygook in medical terms – you're not creating more nerves! What they are talking about is regulating function, and it's a theory; what you may be doing is altering the situation so that the flow of nerve impulses is regulated at a more appropriate level. But I don't know if anyone has gone in and measured the frequency. I'm interested in what the effect of something is and whether it works.

'I wanted to train because I was aware, working both as a GP and in a casualty department, how ineffective many treatments were for back pain. Before starting the training I had some McTimoney treatments, and I was very impressed that the places that the chiropractor was picking up as needing treatment were the places where I felt discomfort. As for the concept of Innate Intelligence, I wish more doctors functioned out of that premise. It wouldn't be "This is what I am doing to you", it would be "We are co-operating to allow the healing aspect of yourself to come into play." To me that makes a lot of sense.'

Another Option

The IPC does not see itself as being in competition with the BCA, but as providing another option. There is a clear difference in its approach to diagnosis and its view of the chiropractor's role, as well as differences in terminology. As far as manipulative techniques are concerned, no comparative studies have been made of the effectiveness of the two methods. Both schools are successful in treating a wide range of musculo-skeletal disorders and some cases of organic disorder. Both have patients whom they can help but not cure, and both admit to having their failures. In some cases IPC practitioners have helped the failed patients of BCA chiropractors and vice versa; just as both IPC and BCA chiropractors have successfully treated the failed patients of osteopaths, while osteopaths have been known to succeed where chiropractic has failed. This leads one to the conclusion that technique alone is not the whole answer to any medical problem. Some manipulators are more skilled than others, whatever technique they use; in some cases, too, the key seems to lie in that mysterious, unscientifically-testable element, the rapport between patient and therapist.

'The basic message is that there are different forms of treatment,' says an IPC chiropractor. 'I'm pretty open-minded; I say, try me, and if it doesn't work you don't have to come again. There is no right or wrong, there is what is right for you.'

CHAPTER THREE

VISITING A CHIROPRACTOR

Choosing a Chiropractor

Most people visit chiropractors on the recommendation of friends. Otherwise, unless your GP is able and willing to refer you, you should apply to one of the chiropractic organizations for a copy of their register or the name and address of your nearest practitioner. Only in this way can you be sure of his or her qualifications. As in other European countries, there are some chiropractors in Britain who are not included on a register, either through choice or through lack of the appropriate qualifications. Some have trained in America or Canada; there are still a few who trained through apprenticeship; and although I have not come across an instance myself, I am told that there are also people calling themselves chiropractors who have not trained anywhere at all.

Chiropractors who have qualified in North America use the initials D.C. (Doctor of Chiropractic) after their names, as do AECC graduates; some, but not all, also use the title 'Doctor'.* McTimoney-trained chiropractors use the initials C.P. (Chiropractic Practitioner, followed by A.I.P.C. or M.I.P.C.); they do not use the title 'Doctor'.

*Different rules apply in different countries. In America it is legal and customary for chiropractors to use the 'Doctor' title. According to *Chiropractic in New Zealand*, New Zealand chiropractors who had qualified in America consequently felt entitled to call themselves 'Doctor', and many of them were doing so in 1979, to the severe irritation of medical doctors. The Commission saw no objection to their using the initials D.C., but felt that use of the word 'Doctor' could be misleading. In Britain, under the Medical Act of 1956 people who are not registered medical practitioners are prohibited from 'wilfully and falsely' using a title which implies that they are so registered, but this does not prohibit an unregistered person from using the title 'Doctor' if they hold a doctor's degree in a non-medical subject, and so long as the public is not misled.

One defect of the freedom with which alternative practitioners practise in Britain is that anyone, including you and me, can put any letters we choose after our names. So it is inadvisable to visit a chiropractor or other manipulator about whom you know nothing unless his name appears on a professional register. There are undoubtedly some individuals outside any of the professional bodies who are skilled manipulators, but there are two problems here. First, they may not be skilled in diagnosis; secondly, the public has no means of distinguishing them from charlatans – other than by trial and error. And, although instances are rare, an error in manipulating the spine can prove irreversible.

If you approach a chiropractor direct you are not obliged to tell your doctor, although McTimoney practitioners prefer you to do so. My own feeling is that if there were more communication between doctors and complementary therapists, there would be fewer misunderstandings and less prejudice on both sides. (And one practical advantage is that if your doctor has already had X-rays taken and is willing for you to take them to your chiropractor, you may avoid having to have further ones taken.)

Visiting a BCA Chiropractor

The first visit is generally devoted to diagnosis, and can last up to an hour if the problem is complex or long-standing. The chiropractor will take a full case history, including all previous accidents or falls, and your medical history, past and present. He or she* will need to know if you are taking medication, as in certain conditions treatment may reduce the dosage requirement (another good reason for communication with doctors). He may also ask about your eating and

*I apologize to women chiropractors if from now on in this section I refer to all chiropractors as 'he' for the sake of easy reading.

working habits and general lifestyle, all of which have a bearing on your health.

He will then give you a physical examination, taking you through a series of movements and other tests to assess your posture and mobility – standing, bending forwards and sideways, and so on. He will then ask you to sit or lie on his treatment table so that he can palpate your spine, gently going over it with his hands to assess muscle tone and the condition of the tissues around the joints. He will look at the comparative length of your legs; although a surprising number of people have slightly irregular leg lengths, discrepancies often indicate that a muscular contraction is distorting the symmetry of the pelvis. (Sometimes a genuinely longer leg has been found, and supplying a lift for the shorter leg can make a lot of difference to a back problem.) He will also test the strength of various muscles; he may include AK tests, but there are also standard tests in a muscle weakness which can indicate where there is an irritated nerve, since the signal sent by the nerve is not strong enough for the muscle to maintain its strength.

The chiropractor is likely to examine the whole of your spine, not just the painful area; since everything in the body's structure interrelates, a problem in one section often has repercussions on others. Equally, if the reason for your visit is not your back but perhaps a knee or elbow joint, the problem may still originate in the spine. Finally, one or two X-rays may be taken; if the chiropractor does not have his own equipment he will arrange for this to be taken by a radiographer before your next visit.

Unless your case is very simple, such as a recent wrench, or an emergency causing acute pain, treatment will probably not begin until your next visit; this will take around fifteen minutes (plus or minus, according to what needs to be done). On your second visit the chiropractor will report to you on the results of your X-rays and explain them to you. He will also tell you how far he thinks he can help you

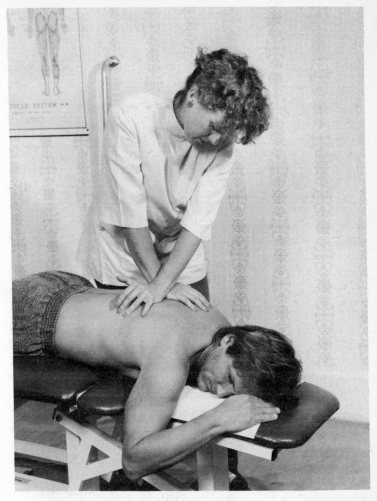

A chiropractor adjusts the thoracic spine

– though at this stage he probably won't be able to tell you precisely how long the full course of treatments will take, since patients react in individual ways. Then he will ask you to strip to your underwear and put on a robe for the treatment itself.

As we have seen, the chiropractor has a whole battery of techniques to choose from, and he will obviously employ those he considers most appropriate to your case. Different techniques may be used at different stages of treatment, particularly when a person has a long-standing problem. Whether manipulation is painful or not depends on a number of factors including the patient's problem and degree of sensitivity, as well as the chiropractor's individual touch. (My own experience of both BCA and McTimoney chiropractic is that they are gentler than I expected, and also gentler than some osteopathic adjustments I have received, but it would be unfair to generalize from this: there seems to be a trend towards gentler techniques in many therapies.) Manipulation of the spine and joints is both a science and an art, and every individual has his own way of handling the body. As people are likely to be in pain to start with, there may be some brief pain during an adjustment – which should be outweighed by the prospect of long-term relief!

Very often, as an adjustment is made, a slight – or even loud – 'click'* is heard. Patients usually assume that this noise is made by a vertebra 'going back into place', and when it occurs it certainly feels as though something has been achieved, but it is not essential to the success of a treatment. During my research for this book I have been politely reproved by more than one BCA chiropractor for referring to backs or joints being 'out', since they regard this as anatomically inaccurate. Vertebrae, they say, don't 'go out' in the first place; in fact the only joints that can move during a spinal adjustment are the facet joints which link the vertebrae, and if they move it is only slightly.

Some chiropractors offer additional facilities, such as

---

*Research carried out by a group at Leeds University suggests that the 'pop' during an adjustment (or occurring spontaneously) is caused by the bursting of a nitrogen bubble in the synovial fluid round the joint as the joint capsule is stretched.

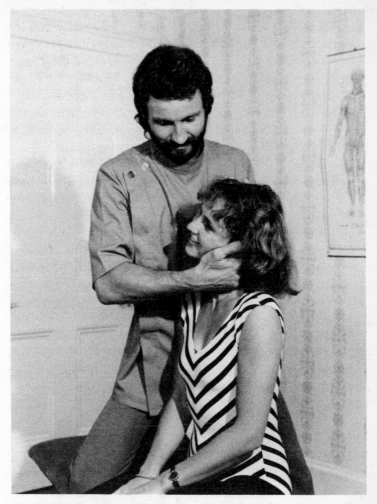

Adjusting the neck doesn't have to be alarming

ultrasound or other mechanical devices, for pain relief, or
traction; those who own them are cautious about over-use,
and others prefer to stick to manual techniques. As one
says: 'Attaching a person to a machine while you go away
and have a cup of tea is not chiropractic.'

McTimoney Treatment

A visit to a McTimoney chiropractor also starts with taking a case history, covering similar questions to those asked by BCA chiropractors, but excluding clinical tests or X-rays; the chiropractor will ask whether you have had a medical diagnosis. Some patients bring X-rays if they already have them, and the chiropractor may arrange for them to be taken if he thinks this essential.

After taking the case history the chiropractor will begin treatment; this lasts between thirty and sixty minutes. The chiropractor checks the whole body from head to toe. 'It's like having a 12,000-mile service of a car,' Stan Harding explains. 'If the wheel of your car is wearing the tyre out, you'll not only replace the tyre, if you've got any sense you'll look at the tracking, the true cause of the problem.' Chiropractors believe the true cause of many dis-eases originates in spinal subluxations or fixations.

This 'whole-body technique' includes palpating and, when appropriate, gently manipulating the skull and face (the jaw is often a site of great tension). Differences in leg length are assessed; both the front and back of the body will be palpated for misalignments, and adjustments made on those joints that require it, chiefly using the very light toggle recoil technique which restores mobility to the joint. The hands and feet will also receive a 'service', whether or not the patient has obvious problems in those areas.

IPC practitioners usually leave a week to ten days between treatments in order to see how the body is adapting; improvements should occur within six treatments, although obviously some cases take longer. 'We start a process of healing,' one of them says. 'It is the body that heals; we are simply trying to help.'

Reactions to Treatment

Chiropractors of both schools usually warn patients after

their first treatment that they may experience reactions of various kinds. One very common occurrence is for patients to feel quite tired. This is a natural result of the relaxation brought about by the relief of pain and tension, and of the effects of spinal adjustment on the nervous system; patients may be advised to rest for a quarter of an hour after treatment, and some need to sleep. A McTimoney chiropractor treated a woman whose neck had been hurt in a car crash four years before; realizing that he had brought about a profound change, he suggested she rest before she went home. She retorted that she had scarcely slept for four years and didn't need to rest. She drove her car nearly as far as the motorway, pulled in to the side and slept for seven hours. Although this is an extreme example, it is worth taking note and not timing a treatment to take place immediately before you plan to do something strenuous or demanding.

Stiffness or soreness may occur in some people for a day or two afterwards, even after a very gentle treatment; occasionally people even experience an increase in pain for a short time, brought about by the unaccustomed stretching of tight muscles as the body readjusts. A good chiropractor will suggest that you telephone him if you are worried by such reactions, or by any other unaccustomed changes in the body – sometimes women experience changes in their menstrual cycle and are glad to be reassured that this is quite normal. Some patients walk out on a euphoric 'high', partly due to the relief of pain, and possibly again to the effects of work on the nervous system.

Of course the most desirable reaction to treatment is that the patient will feel better, but this may not necessarily occur immediately. Although chiropractic deals with body mechanics, bodies are not machines that can be instantly fixed by tightening a screw here or oiling a joint there. The results of any one treatment may take effect over the next few days or even weeks as the body readapts.

How Many Treatments Are Needed?

The spacing and number of treatments must depend on the patient's own needs and the individual chiropractor's approach. McTimoney chiropractor Stan Harding says that a patient who gets better after one session is a bit of a pain, because his friends will come along expecting identical results, whatever their problem. 'We live in a world that wants instant responses, and people want instant healing,' he comments. 'But you have to understand that healing is a process, not a single event. After all, you may have taken years to get into your present condition; it would be reasonable to expect it to take some time to get better.' Some patients are asked to come once or twice a week to begin with; some chiropractors prefer to leave a longer interval between treatments in order to see how the body responds.

The BCA and IPC quote an average of six to ten visits, and the New Zealand report includes the following table:

Number of visits	Percentages of patients
1–3	9
4–6	29
7–9	23
10–12	26
13–15	6
over 15	7

As a rough guide, the older you are and the longer you have had your problem, the more treatments you will need. You and your chiropractor should have a good idea within four to six sessions how far you can be helped.

Chiropractors recognize the interrelationship of different parts of the body. If one segment of the spine is affected, this can throw other segments out of balance; this is referred to as 'compensation'. For example, an asymmetrical pelvis will cause the spine to be slightly tilted; the person then automatically tilts the head in order to look the world straight-on. As the neck muscles become habituated to this tilt, it too can become a built-in problem. Slight scoliosis may occur as well (lateral curves in the spine, producing a kind of 'S' shape). Conversely, a tilt in the neck may, over time, lead to pelvic problems. So the chiropractor, faced with several problem areas, will tend to deal with the most recent problem first, taking some time to reach the original cause. Thus the person who arrives with a lower-back problem may find the chiropractor at some stage treating their neck and even their skull. During this kind of unravelling process – sometimes referred to as 'retracing' – there are times when the patient may feel noticeably worse, or experience a recurrence of symptoms he thought were past and gone; these effects are only temporary, however, and the chiropractor will reassure the patient by explaining what is going on.

As treatments continue, the chiropractor reassesses the patient at every visit; diagnosis is an on-going process. If a patient does not progress as well as expected, he may need to reconsider the course of adjustments originally decided on, or check whether another factor is involved, such as nutrition or an emotional problem. He may well recommend exercises, suggest ways of improving posture, and discuss other factors, such as your working conditions, diet, or level of stress.

Chiropractors are particularly concerned to help patients to help themselves, and of course this demands the patient's cooperation. Stan Harding comments that the people who come to him have to work! 'Some of those referred by doctors are simply not interested in their own health, and then it comes home to me what a hard job doctors have.' By contrast, a hospital worker, the patient of another chiropractor, was delighted to be shown ways of improving her posture and physical habits. 'It puts control back in your own hands, and it works,' she says.

As we have seen, how far a chiropractor advises on

general health varies according to the patient's needs and the chiropractor's interests, but if he feels there is a health problem that he cannot deal with himself he will suggest an appropriate doctor or other therapist. Further X-rays or investigation may be indicated; sometimes these have revealed the beginnings of a growth that was not visible at the first visit, and in such cases patients are referred for medical treatment.

There are always, unfortunately, conditions that are not completely curable, but which can still be greatly helped; the patient may then need to return at regular, though longer, intervals so that the chiropractor can maintain the improvements he has brought about and prevent further deterioration.

Costs

Average charges for chiropractic in Britain in 1986 are £15 for the first consultation and £10 for follow-up visits. The IPC encourages its members not to charge more than £10, but for both the BCA and the IPC charges may vary around the country, and are likely to be higher in London where overheads are higher. X-rays are about £8 a plate, though they will cost more if they have to be taken by an independent radiographer. Compared with the real costs of medical treatment chiropractic fees are not high; even so, some patients find them a problem, particularly if a long course of treatment is required. The fees of one or two BCA chiropractors are recoupable on BUPA or PPP insurance schemes. Most BCA and IPC chiropractors try to find ways of subsidizing the less well-off or of staggering payments for long-term treatment. Although alternative practitioners are often accused of being 'in it for the money' (and as with people in any profession a few of them probably are) the majority actually care about their patients' health.

Does It Work – And Is It Safe?

Chiropractic has not only survived a century of opposition: it has flourished. Clearly, it has something to offer. The majority of patients visit chiropractors initially with back problems, often after orthodox medicine has failed to help them. In this area chiropractic is undoubtedly effective and also undoubtedly safe.

Not all doctors are convinced of these facts; the results of any kind of manipulation are notoriously difficult to assess scientifically, and more research is still needed in this field, particularly in the UK. However, this view is changing. A number of chiropractors have built up good relations with local medical practices who refer patients when appropriate. The public in general believes that conventional medicine is not good at dealing with backs;* while patients are more concerned with their individual back-aches than with statistics, such studies as have been carried out would seem to support their views, including a number of studies by Workmen's Compensation Boards in the USA, and the extremely thorough survey of chiropractic carried out in New Zealand in 1979. Two surveys carried out in Denmark (1963 and 1970), also by a government Commission of Inquiry, indicate that for over-all problems the response rate (from major improvement to total loss of symptoms) is 82 to 85 per cent.

According to the New Zealand Commission's report, published in a highly readable 376-page volume, *Chiropractic in New Zealand*, 'there can be no doubt that chiropractic treatment is effective for musculo-skeletal

---

*Seventy-five per cent of people visiting alternative therapists present with musculo-skeletal problems.

disorders'. On the question of whether spinal manual therapy can influence organic and/or visceral disorders, the Commission was 'satisfied that in some cases this is at least a possibility'. These conclusions were formulated after the Commission had spent nearly two years thoroughly investigating chiropractic in New Zealand and other parts of the world, and hearing the testimony on oath of chiropractors, doctors and patients, elicited by a barrister skilled in cross-examination.

The Commission also concluded that chiropractic is 'remarkably safe', and supported the use of X-rays as a safeguard against misdiagnosis. The safety of chiropractic is also indicated by the fact that in England the Medical Research Council has authorized trials to be carried out to compare the relative effectiveness of chiropractic and hospital out-patient treatment.

No physical treatment is 100 per cent safe. Chiropractors are human; they do make mistakes, and are very open about admitting this, though their mistakes are not usually of a disastrous nature. (Interestingly, one BCA practitioner decided to take up the profession five years after his mother had been cured and two years after his father had been damaged by the same somewhat elderly chiropractor! Talking with the chiropractor concerned, he became fascinated by the fact that although the public assumes that medicine has all the answers, the action of drugs, for instance, is not fully understood and there is a great deal yet to be learned about the human body. Chiropractic appealed to his fascination with discovery.)

If accidents do occur, the BCA and IPC both have complaints procedures and disciplinary committees, at least providing the patient with some form of come-back. When a patient is damaged by an alternative therapist who does not belong to a professional body, it is always possible to sue the therapist, but one cannot sue him for more than he has. Where professions are properly organized, as in the case of chiropractic, practitioners are covered by professional insurance schemes. Another indication of the relative safety of chiropractic is the fact that the cost of annual insurance against legal liability in 1986 was under £50 for chiropractors, in contrast with that for the medical profession, which was £288.

In fact most complaints don't reach the point of litigation. Complaints are sometimes received from patients who are not getting better; a cure is of course something no chiropractor can guarantee, and when this kind of case has been investigated the chiropractor will only be disciplined if he is also considered to have behaved unethically. One was removed from the BCA register for continuing to treat a patient for ten years without making her better; she then went to another therapist who brought about a rapid recovery. Such instances are very rare. There is a high standard of ethics among chiropractors, and one who has not succeeded in making a patient better will usually acknowledge this and refer the patient to a colleague who may be more successful.

PART THREE

WHAT CAN CHIROPRACTIC TREAT?

CHAPTER ONE

THE PROBLEM OF BACK PAIN

It is hardly surprising that the majority of chiropractic patients arrive with back pain: it is a nationwide problem – one that affects all industrialized countries, in fact. Its scale is indicated by the latest statistics, or, rather, estimates, since accurate figures are hard to establish. Between 80 and 100 per cent of the British population are believed to experience back pain at some stage in life. According to the Office of Health Economics,* in one year at least 22,900,000 episodes are experienced in the population of the UK as a whole; of these only about 2,200,000 sufferers consult general practitioners, which is still three times the number attributable to coronary heart disease. Some 330,000 are then referred to specialists, 63,000 of whom enter hospitals as in-patients, and something under 10,000 will be given surgery.

The estimated cost of back pain to the NHS in 1982 was £156.1 million. Lost to industry were 33.3 million days of working time – exceeding the losses attributable to both coronary heart disease and bronchitis, and more than six times the number of working days lost through industrial stoppages in 1982. Social security payments resulting from these amounted to an estimated total of £193 million in 1982–3.

It is impossible to estimate the cost to the individual;

*Back Pain, Office of Health Economics, London, 1985.

apart from loss of work and payment for analgesics and special aids, the physical and emotional costs cannot be quantified. How do you measure difficulty in daily dressing, cooking, or getting out of the house? Or the wearing effects of on-going pain, both on sufferers and their families?

So what makes the spine so particularly vulnerable?

The Structure of the Spine

The spine has been described as a marvel of engineering. It consists of twenty-four vertebrae, bone segments joined together by muscles and ligaments. It is divided into five main regions: there are seven cervical vertebrae in the neck, twelve thoracic vertebrae in the back of the chest and five lumbar vertebrae in the low back. Below the lumbar region is the sacrum at the back of the hip bones, a solid, shield-like piece of bone consisting of five sacral vertebrae virtually fused together. Finally comes the coccyx – the remnants of a tail – with three to five coccygeal vertebrae, which may be either separate or fused.

Each vertebra consists of an oval-shaped main body, from which protuberances called bony processes project backwards and sideways for the attachment of muscles and ligaments. One, the spinous process, creates the 'knob' which can be felt through the skin of the back. The articular and transverse processes jutting from the sides link neatly in with those of the vertebrae above and below, to form facet joints. These are synovial joints, like other joints of the body; that is, they have a lining called a synovium, which keeps the joint lubricated with synovial fluid, and are surrounded by a protective capsule.

Other synovial joints in the spine are the atlanto-occipital joint, joining the first cervical vertebra to the part of the skull called the occiput, and the two sacroiliac joints where

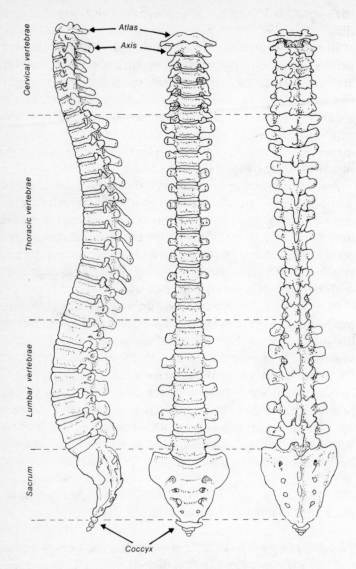

The spinal column – a marvel of engineering

the sacrum is joined to the hip bones at the area called the ilia.

Between the vertebrae lie the discs; they are not, as some people imagine, separate washers which can slip out, but are continuous with the vertebrae, so that the spine forms a flexible rod. Discs consist of an outer ring of cartilage surrounding a softer, jelly-like centre; they have no blood supply and there are some nerve endings in the outer perimeter only. They act as shock-absorbers, changing shape, rather like cushions, as the spine bends.

As well as holding the body up, the spine has the important function of protecting the spinal cord, which emerges from the brain and runs through a canal formed by arches between the main body of the vertebrae and the bony processes. The brain and spinal cord form the central nervous system; they are encased in a tough sheath called a dura, within which they are bathed in cerebro-spinal fluid.

All the way down the spine thirty-one pairs of spinal nerves branch out from the spinal cord to other parts of the body, through gaps between the vertebrae called the intervertebral foramina. These nerves carry messages to and from the brain to different parts of the body; the brain issues instructions – to move, to relax, and so on – and receives messages of pain and other sensations. They link up with the autonomic nervous system, which controls automatic bodily functions like digestion, regulation of heartbeat and blood pressure.

Pain and the Nervous System

Looking at this structure, it is clear that the nerves leaving the spine are susceptible to any abnormal pressure from a joint or disc, which will cause pain. Pain is valuable, in that it tells the body that something is wrong, and the person experiencing pain should take note of it. Back pain indicates that there is pressure on or irritation of a nerve, either as it leaves the spine or elsewhere in the body, and to remove it necessitates tracing and removing the cause. When the cause does not lie in the superficial muscles and ligaments, however, back pain becomes very difficult to diagnose, especially since the spine cannot readily be opened up and examined. Pain may be felt without any obvious signs showing up on an X-ray; on X-rays, for instance, bones are visible, but the discs are only seen as spaces, so disc problems require skilled diagnosis.

Actual pressure on nerves does not occur that often; pain often comes from irritated nerves in joint capsules, or muscles and ligaments around a joint. The source is not always easy to find; pain from around the synovial joints is not very clearly located, and from the surface of the inter-vertebral disc it feels diffuse. Also, the more irritation there is in these pain-sensitive structures, the more distant the pain is likely to become, and the sufferer experiences what is called 'referred pain'. Thus pain originating in certain parts of the back may be felt in the legs, arms, abdomen, chest or even the head.

This is where specialists like chiropractors come in with their knowledge of the spine and nervous system, and skill at detecting very small abnormalities in the joints; the type of pain experienced also gives them information, for example, as to whether a nerve is irritated or inflamed, and also whether the pain is of mechanical origin or has a non-physiological cause such as anxiety.

What Goes Wrong with Backs

Most cases of back-ache are due to strains in the complex system of muscles, ligaments and tendons attached to the spine, rather than to any serious disease or condition, and may include muscle spasm, and pressure on a joint. Medical causes, including inflammatory conditions (such as rheumatoid arthritis and ankylosing spondylitis), cancer and metabolic disorders, are involved only in about 1 to 2 per cent of back-pain cases. Lower-back pain, the commonest back pain of all, is often loosely described as 'lumbago'; this simply means a pain in the lumbar region, and it may stem from a variety of causes. The famous 'slipped disc' only accounts for about 5 to 7 per cent of all low-back pain. (Some doctors incorrectly tell patients that they have a 'slipped disc' in order to provide them with a label for their pain.) Other causes are strains in muscles and ligaments, or joints subluxated or fixated through accident, congenital malformation, sudden unskilful movements or, very often, poor posture or habits of physical or emotional tension.

Long-term stress overworks the adrenal glands which depletes the muscles of vital minerals. (Poor nutrition can have a similar effect.) When this is combined with physical tension muscles may go into spasm, pulling the sacrum out of its proper position. Even more commonly, stress is manifested in the shoulder muscles and the neck.

'I think the reason many people have bad backs is because they're so floppy!' comments the wife of an orthopaedic surgeon. 'Floppiness' is encouraged by much modern furniture design, as well as by the fact that today many people's work involves sitting for long hours. In fact, says George Walker, sitting at school desks for years is a cause of degenerative change in the discs of the young. The natural resting posture for human beings is squatting, which allows the weight to be supported by the thighs and keeps the spine long and the disc spaces open. Sitting, particularly slumping, in low chairs can weaken lower-back muscles and compress the discs in the lower back; this compression squeezes them dry of moisture, depriving them of nutrition and making them vulnerable to damage. Discs can also be damaged by lifting heavy weights incorrectly (a

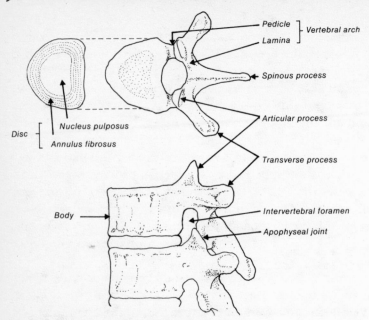

Pedicle ⎤
Lamina ⎦ Vertebral arch

Spinous process

Articular process

Transverse process

Disc ⎡ Nucleus pulposus
⎣ Annulus fibrosus

Body

Intervertebral foramen

Apophyseal joint

Thoracic vertebrae and intervertebral disc

common occurrence among unskilled manual workers), and over-exertion at sports or dancing. Once damaged, the mis-named 'slipped disc' is more likely to occur.

'Slipped Disc'

As mentioned above, discs do not slip out of place; they can't. But they can herniate, and the correct name for the condition is 'disc herniation' or 'disc prolapse'. It does not occur in healthy, undamaged discs; but once a disc has been damaged the prolapse itself can be caused by a fall, twisting, heavy lifting, or just bending to pick something up.

What happens is that the weakened fibrous exterior allows the soft centre of the disc to bulge outwards. This may put pressure on the nerve root as it emerges through the intervertebral foramen. The nerve root may become inflamed, and is sometimes compressed, causing the

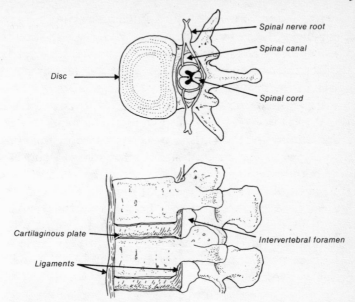

Spinal nerve root

Spinal canal

Disc

Spinal cord

Cartilaginous plate

Intervertebral foramen

Ligaments

Vertebrae of the lumbar spine

sufferer acute pain. Inflammation can cause back pain or sciatic pain in the legs, depending on whether the inflammatory change is affecting the tissues of the spine, the nerve root, or both.

Sciatica

Sciatica is a symptom, not a disease or malfunction in itself. It is caused by mechanical irritation of the sciatic nerve, which originates in the lower back with branches extending down the leg to the toes. It may affect one or both legs, giving rise to searing pain, numbness, disturbed circulation, tingling in the feet and even partial paralysis. The cause of all sciatica is to be found in the lower back, though only 5 per cent of cases are associated with 'slipped discs'.

Osteoarthritis

Osteoarthritis is another misnomer where the spine is

concerned, since arthritis means inflammation of a joint. The bone growth, or calcification, which occurs as the spine ages is not an inflammatory condition. More correctly called arthrosis or spondylosis, it is a natural development, akin to thickening of the skin on the soles of the feet. It occurs in response to wear and tear, usually starting from the age of forty onwards, although it can happen even earlier. In the spine it tends to be present at more than one level, generally the cervical and lumbar regions, and can affect both the synovial joints and the discs. As the spine ages the discs become thinner and more fibrous, and the cartilage between the joints may begin to wear away. The vertebrae become thicker and may grow bony spurs called osteophytes. Many people have 'osteoarthritis' of the spine with no pain at all, though pain may occur when a thickened joint or osteophytes intrude on nerves.

Other Back Problems

These can develop from bad postural habits and tension. For instance, pelvic problems are very common, often arising from long-term habits such as always sitting slightly twisted to type from documents placed on the left, always standing with the weight on one leg, or always carrying heavy objects on the same side. It can occur in runners who constantly run in the same direction round a track. Repetition of these habits can cause the muscles to stretch on one side and shorten on the other, so that over time the condition becomes permanent.

The pelvis can also be pulled out of alignment by accidents or sudden movements – sneezing while lifting, for instance, may give rise to muscle spasm in one hip, if there is a weakness there to start with.

Other problems may have quite subtle causes, needing expert and experienced diagnosis – which they don't always get. Most doctors are not well trained in examining the spine, and to orthopaedic surgeons, who are dealing in 'crisis care', these subtleties may seem unimportant.

Conventional Treatment of Back Pain

By far the majority of back pain is in fact 'self-limiting'; that is, with rest and care the system will heal itself within two to six weeks. It is when pain continues that people generally visit the doctor's surgery.

'Rest and Pills'

The GP, unless he practises manipulation himself or is sold on the idea of chiropractic, will probably prescribe rest and pain-killers – which the patient may already have prescribed for himself. Rest can certainly help the body to heal itself – though too much may weaken the muscles. There is a place for drugs used short-term; by relieving pain they reduce muscle spasm, and thus aid healing by allowing a normal blood supply to return to the joint. Cortisone and other injections can sometimes prove effective, too.

'Pills' range from the simple aspirin to a variety of anti-inflammatory drugs: the dangers of some of these – such as causing internal bleeding – have been well publicized lately, causing anxiety among doctors as well as patients. In addition, a surgeon points out, removing pain and swelling actually does the joint no good, because it also reduces the blood supply which the joint needs to repair itself; at the same time, removing the pain may encourage the person to over-use that joint and damage it further.

Even when doctors give their patients a physical examination the source of the pain, as we have seen, may be far from obvious. As a result patients are all too often labelled as 'neurotic' and are prescribed tranquillizers. Pain may certainly be caused or exacerbated by emotional or psychological problems; that doesn't make it any less real. If stress has created a mechanical problem, physical treatment is needed.

If he is convinced that something is mechanically wrong the GP will refer the patient to a hospital consultant, rheumatologist or orthopaedic surgeon, or possibly direct to a physiotherapist.

Physiotherapy

The role of physiotherapists has expanded of late; they form an independent profession, many of whose members work in private practice and can be approached without a doctor's referral. Within the NHS they now have responsibility for assessing what treatment patients need (this used not to be the case). However, traditionally their treatment is prescribed by the consultant in charge, and they are not all acting with full autonomy as yet.

They are all trained in basic manipulative techniques, and some go on to take further training in manipulation. Their training and manipulative ability varies considerably, however; many simply use mobilization, that is gently moving a joint within its normal range, rather than adjustment, and the adjustments they carry out may be general rather than specific. They can certainly help a number of patients – in fact almost any kind of manipulation will help a proportion of people. However, others may be left unimproved. Physiotherapists agree that there is room for different forms of manipulation, some suiting particular patients better than others.

Other treatments include traction, in which apparatus is used to stretch the spine, thereby relieving pressure on the discs; there is some doubt as to its long-term benefits. Corsets or belts may be prescribed which can relieve pain by supporting the weak area of the back, but of course they will not strengthen the muscles themselves.

Physiotherapists also have a wide range of equipment for relieving pain, improving blood supply and helping tissues to regenerate, including ultrasound and short-wave treatment, and transcutaneous nerve stimulators. A method currently being researched is the application of electromagnetic waves, though it is too early for its results to be reliably evaluated.

An extremely important aspect of care which physiotherapists share with chiropractors is ergonomics, the study of how people use their bodies in carrying out their daily activities. As well as being prescribed remedial exercises, patients are re-educated in how to sit, stand, bend, lift, type, and so on with least damage and pain to the spine. (It would surely improve the nation's health and the NHS economy if ergonomics were included in school curricula.)

Acupuncture and Hypnotherapy

These are offered in some hospitals for patients with intractable pain. However, it is rare for them to bring about permanent relief, and they cannot alter structural damage. They might do more good if they were used earlier. An acupuncturist working in a hospital pain clinic complains that by the time people reach her many have been in pain for years; in addition, they are allocated to have acupuncture rather than choosing it themselves, and this can affect their responses.

Surgery

Surgery tends to be a last resort. It can achieve excellent results, but it is believed to have a failure rate of 10 to 15 per cent and long-term side-effects. Orthopaedic surgeons operate on only about one in twenty of the patients referred to them, and may first try other treatments, including those mentioned above.

One of the most common spinal operations is laminectomy – treatment of a 'slipped disc'. This involves cutting a window through the bones of the spine in order to reach the disc. Formerly the whole disc might be removed, leaving

patients with no 'shock-absorbers' between the vertebrae;
the usual surgical procedure nowadays is to cut through
part of the hard exterior of the disc and remove only the
offending soft centre which is bulging out. This operation
is usually carried out when the back-ache is accompanied
by sciatica. Unfortunately, while relieving sciatica, it often
still leaves people with low-back pain.

Spinal fusion sometimes follows a laminectomy, or may
be carried out when extreme osteoarthritis is causing pain,
either in the lumbar region or in the neck when pain is
going down the upper arm. It consists of fusing two vertebrae together by laying down a bone graft, usually from
the hip bone. This creates rigidity in that area of the spine –
indeed the aim of the operation is to stiffen that section; but
chiropractors have found that as a result the vertebrae
above and below the stiffened area become hypermobile
and overworked in order to compensate; after a while this
leads to further problems and pain.

Orthopaedic surgeons also manipulate joints, generally –
though not always – under anaesthetic, and often quite successfully. Some experts point out that since a correctly performed manipulation should not be painful anaesthesia
should be unnecessary. Also, says a pro-chiropractic surgeon, apart from the slight risk entailed by anaesthetics, it is
easier and quicker for a patient to walk into a chiropractor's
clinic and walk out again half an hour later!

The Chiropractic Alternative

The majority of chiropractors have taken up their profession because they have seen that chiropractic can help
people even when all else has failed, and have often been
successfully treated themselves. Obviously, they do not see
those who are happy with the medical treatment they have
received and grateful to physiotherapists and surgeons, and

I would not wish to suggest that all medical treatment is unsympathetic or unsatisfactory. But it is both sad and wasteful that so many people have to go through the 'all else' – the slow progression from doctor, to hospital, to surgeon and possibly to surgery (with waiting lists at each stage), when they could be relieved of pain and further deterioration could be prevented at a much earlier point.

'Chiropractic manipulation seems to make sense to me,' says the surgeon quoted above. 'So many people are benefited by it. After all, chiropractors have four or five years studying the spine, they should know something! Some of their ideas might be crazy, but the bulk of what they are presenting is good therapy.' And another: 'There are a lot of conditions, of the spine particularly, which are not bad enough to warrant operative treatment; they may be painful, but all you really want is a mechanical adjustment.' But by the time they reach chiropractors many people have had recurrent pain for years; muscles have become fixed, joints have degenerated – and so has the patient's over-all well-being. Pain takes it out of you.

CHAPTER TWO

CHIROPRACTIC TREATMENT

OF BACK PAIN

At what stage should you consider going to a chiropractor? Since a high proportion of back-aches get better on their own in a few weeks some members of the medical profession are sceptical about the value of manipulation, feeling that osteopaths and chiropractors take the credit for cures that would have happened naturally in time. However, many people suffer for months or years before visiting a chiropractor; there is a danger of dismissing recurrent back-ache as unimportant and only belatedly waking up to the fact that one has developed a chronic problem. So if a back-ache doesn't clear up quickly, or tends to return, it is wise to seek prompt treatment. It is also sensible to seek expert advice after a heavy fall or sudden sprain or strain, even if nothing is broken; if some biomechanical damage has been done you may be unaware of it until you develop sciatica five years later. An early check-up can prevent later suffering.

'Very rarely do patients come and see us until the condition has been indwelling for over nine months,' says George Walker. 'Once someone has had a condition for that long and it's recurring, it needs thorough investigation, including X-rays, to establish whether there's any damage, congenital weakness or disease.' There are certain conditions that most chiropractors will not attempt to treat, including inflammatory diseases, cancer of the spine or internal organs, and some congenital conditions. Which still leaves a lot of problems that can be helped.

For many people the advantages of going to an expert

outweigh having to pay for treatment. These include not only expertise, but the fact that one can be seen speedily and will then be given the time, attention and support of one individual. Trained and experienced in examining and treating the spine, the chiropractor is often able to pinpoint the cause of 'undiagnosed' problems. 'The joy of being told it is *this* that's wrong with you, and what is causing it, and what the chiropractor thinks he can do for you! It's such a relief!' enthuses one cured patient. Another joy is the relief of pain, which – depending of course on the problem – can sometimes be immediate.

The mechanism by which manipulation relieves pain is called the 'gate-control theory of pain'. The joints throughout the body contain cells called mechanoceptors, which register movement; stimulating these produces a hormone called an endorphin, which blocks the path through which the message of pain is carried to the brain. Rubbing a banged knee or elbow is an instinctive reaction which produces a similar pain-relieving effect, and is the reason why massage can be so comforting. Endorphins in the cerebrospinal fluid are also associated with states of mental 'high' (they are known as the body's own morphine), and so perhaps account for the sense of euphoria which some people feel after treatment. There is also a theory that pain relief occurs by means of other neurotransmitters within the spinal cord, and there is more to be learned, but it is scientifically accepted that adjustment can and does relieve pain.

What is not scientifically proven is exactly what else occurs during an adjustment, which is why some medical people are still sceptical about manipulation, particularly when chiropractors don't use the same language as doctors – even doctors who manipulate. Dr John Paterson, co-author of *An Introduction to Medical Manipulation*, says: 'We talk about the painful vertebral segmental disorder, which is exactly true: it's painful, it's segmental in site, and there is a disorder in that it's not working properly. In time we hope we will have clear evidence to show whether we are putting a bone back in place or not; as yet, we don't know.'

It is currently impossible, as a surgeon points out, to look inside the spine of a live, conscious person to find out exactly what's going on in there; and no immediate change may be seen on before-and-after X-rays. As we have seen, chiropractors say that they are restoring function to the joints. 'We may be treating minimal movements,' says a chiropractor, 'but they can have gross effects on the function of the spine, preventing you from bending sideways or making it painful to sit.' For example, the facet joints which should glide easily over each other may be locked, owing to muscle sprain or spasm, which can irritate the nerve as it comes out from between the joints. Chiropractic treatment can free these joints, with no change being shown on an X-ray. But both chiropractors and patients know that a change has been made, and here it is experience, not theory, that counts. 'Some doctors say you can't move the sacro-iliac joint,' says James Rousseau. 'But I know I can – I've felt it move!'

So let us look at some of the changes that chiropractic can bring about – bearing in mind that each person has individual problems, and is treated individually.

'Slipped Disc'

Disc injury is most serious in the young, since their discs contain a lot of fluid, making the bulge of the prolapse very large. Chiropractic treatment in such cases needs to be carried out with enormous care. Bladder and bowel obstruction can result from trapped nerves in the spine, in which case surgery may be the only solution.

If possible, chiropractors prefer to regard surgery as a last resort, because of its potential after-effects. Most disc problems occur between the ages of thirty and fifty, when

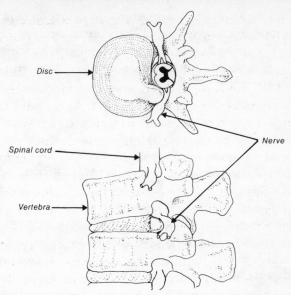

A prolapsed disc. Discs don't slip, but they can bulge, causing pain by pressing against a spinal nerve

they are less serious than in the young, and some middle-aged people are able to go to a chiropractor crippled with a disc prolapse and after a series of treatments walk happily out. With age, discs tend to shrink, becoming narrower, drier and more fibrous, which makes manipulation much easier. Bulging discs can't be pushed back in; treatment consists of creating a wider space between the vertebrae each side, allowing it to slip back into place. (The same principle is applied in traction.)

The speed of cure will depend on the individual case. Sometimes months of treatment may be needed, with improvement taking place only gradually. The chiropractor will have some idea at the start when a cure may be slow; 'I warn these patients that they may get very despondent,' says one. This is where a good relationship between therapist and patient is invaluable.

Expertise is also vitally important. Some more general-ized manipulative techniques include bending or twisting the body, which can further damage the disc. Chiropractic, with its very specific adjustments, is one of the safest forms of treatment.

Sciatica

Only a small proportion of cases of sciatica are caused by disc prolapse. Chiropractic treatment is aimed at finding out exactly where and how the sciatic nerve root is being irritated and relieving it by correct adjustment.

Pelvis Problems

Like 'putting your back out', the phrase 'putting your pelvis out' is deplored by BCA chiropractors, who like to be anatomically accurate. Some prefer to define the prob-lem more specifically as a 'torqued pelvis'. (The correct term is in fact 'X-axis pelvic rotation'.) Whatever you call it, an asymmetrically positioned pelvis is extremely common, and can lead to a variety of aches and pains in the lower back. 'Many of the people I see are a shambles below the waistline,' says Bronwen Herbertson. 'The spine may look pretty good but the pelvis, sacrum and the legs gener-ally aren't well looked after in my terms. If they were, I think many of those "insoluble" problems would not be insoluble any more. Pelvis problems are so common; among other things they can make close relationships uncomfortable if not downright impossible. I've treated numbers of people who've said, "Thank you, my back-ache's gone completely, and I can make love now!"'

Restoring the pelvis to its correct function may take a good number of treatments. Incidentally, at least one orthopaedic surgeon believes that chiropractors and osteo-paths may be 'spinning a yarn' to patients when they ask them to come for several treatments. He says: 'I use an osteopathic technique called rotational manipulation, but I'd only do it once. People walk in with real pain in the spine, with this funny tilted pelvis, and they walk out of the surgery and they've lost their tilt and they're great. But if they don't come straight then, no amount of manipulation is going to cure them.'

This is not the experience of chiropractors and their patients. It is certainly possible to straighten the pelvis in one manipulation; but very often the condition has built up over a period of months or years, affecting the whole balance of the spine and back muscles. It takes time not only to manipulate the relevant areas, but for the body to re-learn its correct balance. As well as receiving manipula-tive treatment, patients can hasten their healing by follow-ing their chiropractor's guidance as to posture, seating arrangements, body use and exercise. This may involve altering the habits of years.

Ankylosing Spondylitis

This auto-immune disease usually occurs in men in their early thirties, occasionally affecting young women too. It starts as a painful inflammatory condition, followed by an increasing tendency for the vertebrae to fuse together. If left untreated, the spine becomes both curved and com-pletely solid – ankylosed. Manipulation is generally inad-visable during the inflammatory stage, but when it reaches the 'cold' stage gentle chiropractic treatment can help to maintain flexibility in the joints, and prevent the ligaments and muscles from shortening and holding the joints tightly. In some patients, though not all, the disease has been halted during treatment. One man, now sixty, developed the condition in his thirties; through visiting a chiropractor about once a month he has benefited a great deal and is still able to lead an active life, including pursuing his hobby of fishing.

After-effects of Injury

Many people suffer unnecessarily for years after back injuries. One quite dramatic case is cited in *Chiropractic in New Zealand*. Mr V. had a car accident in 1933. For ten years afterwards he spent long periods in bed and was at one time partially paralysed. Pain-relieving pills and several courses of physiotherapy did little good; eventually he went to a chiropractor and was greatly helped. As he has a physically active career – and in 1975 built his own house – he has continued to have maintenance treatment once a month.

Another New Zealand case is that of a farmer who around 1949 was prescribed bone fusion following a back injury. A friend persuaded him to go to a chiropractor; after a course of treatments the effects of his injury disappeared and he needed no further treatment. Thirty years later, at seventy-seven, he was in excellent health, farming, shearing sheep and taking part in axemen's competitions!

In England Mrs E. injured her back in two bad falls within a year; the doctor's only remedy was pain-killers. Taking a sedentary office job added to her pain, and brought on sciatica and increased stiffness. When more pain-killers proved ineffective she was sent for an X-ray, which showed arthritis in the spine as a result of the injuries. She was told that there was no remedy except to continue taking drugs, which she disliked. It was another doctor, a woman, who suggested that she should try chiropractic, which she had never heard of. It took a year of almost weekly visits for her to reach the stage where she could live a normal life, but she regards the results as 'miraculous'.

After-effects of Surgery

Surgery does not always completely remove pain, and can leave the back weakened. The joints above a fused section of the spine tend to become hypermobile, causing further pain; this can be treated preventatively by chiropractic.

Alison Gordon-Creed, now at twenty-five a chiropractor herself, started having sciatic symptoms at the age of seventeen, probably as a result of overdoing gymnastics and dance as a child. She says: 'Three orthodox doctors could find nothing on X-rays and told me not to worry, I was young and it would go away. It didn't. I was living in America at the time, and went to a chiropractor there who provided temporary relief, but when I stopped going weekly it came back. For two and a half years I had sciatica down both legs, and became virtually paralysed. I ended up having a laminectomy to treat two ruptured discs. The hospital told me nothing about the after-effects, but when I insisted on knowing they said I would only ever swim or walk, and would get calcification of the joints within two years. The back pain returned, and when I came to England taking a secretarial job aggravated it. Then a friend recommended a McTimoney chiropractor and I went along. I thought it was a joke, because the treatment was completely different from what I'd been used to anywhere – I could hardly feel it, and I thought this isn't any good! He's just flapping his hands about! But the next day, though my muscles felt like I'd had a good workout in the gym, I was totally pain-free with no neck problems, headache or backache. After a course of treatments, there's nothing I can't do. I've been trekking in the Himalayas, and have qualified as a McTimoney chiropractor. Since my work involves bending over people all day and there are bits missing in my back, I have treatment every two or three months. And I haven't developed any calcification.'

As a result of her own experience, Alison is very conscious of the importance of preventative action. She carefully observes how her patients stand and sit, and makes them aware that quite small changes of posture can relieve pain. 'If you can be free of pain 80 per cent of the time, it gives the body a chance to heal,' she says.

Failed Back Surgery

When back surgery fails, it does so with a vengeance. At a BCA clinic I met two patients, now married to each other, both crippled in their early forties after successive operations, including spinal fusions which went wrong. Both husband and wife felt angry that they had not been told of the possible consequences of the many operations they had undergone, and let down by the lack of after-care available within the NHS system to help them adjust to a lifetime of pain. At one point the husband was even sent to a psychiatric hospital as a result of his severe depression, which contributed to the break-up of his first marriage. 'But I am not a mental case,' he points out. 'I am a person who has suffered constant chronic pain for seven years, seven major surgical operations on my spine, and constant optimistic reassurances of their success from all concerned. I also have serious problems with the blood veins at the bottom of my spine which make it practically impossible for me to survive any operation to relieve the pain.' His wife, a former nurse, is also in constant pain.

What can a chiropractor do for people like this? The clock cannot be put back to restore their damaged spines. Treatment has enabled the husband to leave his wheelchair and walk on two sticks. In addition, the chiropractor diagnosed that he had a malfunctioning lower bowel (a not infrequent problem after back operations) which was adding to his despondency by creating a permanent feeling of unwellness; this is now being treated with regular colonic irrigation. Chiropractic cannot completely remove his pain, or his wife's, but it can prevent their conditions from deteriorating further. Most importantly, they no longer feel deserted. The chiropractor understands the mental effects of chronic pain; he is not just a 'back doctor': he is also counsellor, support, social worker and friend.

It requires experience and a certain attitude to take on cases of this kind, and not every chiropractor may be willing and able to give this kind of support. Those who can seem to be filling a role that is, unfortunately, rarely filled in health care in Britain.

Osteoarthritis

As we have seen, calcification of the vertebrae is more properly called arthrosis or spondylosis, but it is common for doctors to call it arthritis, a word that patients understand – and on which they may also put the worst interpretation. Ian Hutchinson is a chiropractor who currently represents the BCA on the Back Pain Association council. He says: 'If you can get one message across, it is that in the spine arthritis is really not as important as in other joints, such as the hips. Too often people are sent for an X-ray and the report of osteoarthritis comes back to the GP who doesn't actually see the X-ray. It's difficult in a report to describe the degree of it, and very often it's not clinically significant at all. But just the mention of it conjures up being crippled and ending up in a wheelchair! Even if it's quite pronounced it can still be helped by manipulation of the spine. It does depend where you've got it and to what extent. But no end of patients are told they've got arthritis and have got to live with it, and in most cases that's actually wrong, because we can still help them.'

Surgery may be the only answer for certain cases, and a chiropractor can judge when it is necessary. But a large number of people can be helped. Chiropractic will not remove the calcification, but it will relieve pain, increase the blood supply to the joints, and help the patient to retain mobility.

Problems of Old Age

Old age should not be a barrier to seeking chiropractic help, whether for osteoarthritis or for other conditions. With age, the bones tend to lose calcium and become more brittle, particularly in women; this condition, called *osteoporosis*, is the reason why it is so easy for elderly people to fracture bones.* Osteoporosis does not cause pain in itself, but as bone shrinks the spine shortens, and episodes of pain may occur as the muscles adapt. Sometimes a vertebra can fracture of its own accord, through a kind of 'metal fatigue'; the chiropractor can increase mobility and relieve pain by treating the soft tissues around it.

Old people are too often told that they must live with their pain, or are issued with pain-killers they would prefer not to take, when in fact they could be helped by gentle chiropractic treatment. One woman, now seventy-nine, had suffered many years with low-back, neck and general spinal pain; doctors and specialists prescribed pain-killers, which did little for her. She finally went to a woman chiropractor belonging to the BCA who has been working on her for four years, using soft-tissue techniques only – gently and

---

*Osteoporosis may occur earlier in people who have to adopt a low-fat diet, which deprives the body of calcium; as a preventative measure for such people and for women at and after the menopause, some chiropractors recommend taking supplements Vitamin C and calcium (the latter can be bought combined with Vitamin D, which helps the body to absorb it).

painlessly massaging the muscles without manipulating the painful joints. Since her fourth treatment her condition has been stable; she feels 'half her age' and is still very active.

Another seventy-nine-year-old, Mrs Peake, had been 'under osteopaths for fifteen years' following a 'slipped disc'. The first one she went to was very helpful, but unfortunately he died, and his successors were less effective. Her condition deteriorated, and she was 'crawling about on two sticks' when she went to see a woman McTimoney chiropractor. 'It was completely different from osteopathy, it didn't hurt at all,' she reports. 'After six or seven treatments, I could walk about again. I continued going weekly for two months, really for toning up; I walk the dog in the park, and have no pain at all now. It's miraculous!'

Chiropractic for the Seriously Ill

There are certain diseases, such as cancer and multiple sclerosis, which no British chiropractor would claim to treat, let alone cure. (Some American chiropractors are bolder in this respect!) However, this should not mean that a seriously ill person should be denied treatment for back problems, and possibly some relief of pain.

It must be rare for someone to start seeing a chiropractor after developing cancer, but some cancer sufferers who are already chiropractic patients do continue to see their practitioners, and find this helpful. While manipulating a person with a spinal tumour is generally contra-indicated (in certain cases very gentle treatment may be appropriate), there are other types of cancer in which gentle spinal adjustment may help to provide relief from pain, as well as from general tension and anxiety. As we have seen, manipulation can help to relieve pain through the action of the nervous system; in addition, many cancer patients have

negative feelings towards their bodies, and the psychological comfort of being caringly touched should not be
underestimated.

Multiple sclerosis sufferers can develop a number of back
and joint problems, since the disease weakens the muscles
that hold the joints together, and quite a few MS patients
find chiropractic helpful in this respect, There are other
conditions, such as the effects of a stroke, which chiropractors will not aim to cure, but they may be able to maintain
the spine and joints in a better condition than would otherwise be the case.

In such cases it is obviously desirable for the chiropractor
to be in communication with the patient's medical advisers.

Cure – or Maintenance?

People sometimes approach alternative or complementary
medicine with the hope that the practitioner is going to
wave some magic, non-medical wand that will make them
better overnight. Unfortunately, life isn't like that. Chiropractic is based on sound mechanical principles, which include the fact that some damage cannot be undone, and that
some conditions will inevitably take a long time to treat. As
we have seen, the body may have compensated for an
original subluxation, requiring the re-balancing of different
areas of the spine.

In addition, the body actually learns habits of pain.
When pain continues over a period of time, it establishes a
kind of pattern in the nervous system, which makes it more
difficult to get rid of; this is called the *law of facilitation*.
The process is like creating a footpath across a field; the
first person to walk across the grass will make no long-term
impact, but years of ramblers walking the same route will
leave their mark. A single manipulation can break the cycle

of pain, but if the pain-path has become well established it will recur. The law of facilitation also means that even after treatment pain can recur more easily under a stimulus, such as stress or over-exertion, which might not affect someone else.

As well as pain habits, the body tends to acquire individual mechanical habits, which chiropractors call *fixation*; under stress of any kind it is easy to slip back into a particular pattern. So once treatment is complete it is important to remain aware of postural habits and keep up preventative exercises. Some chiropractors recommend patients to learn the Alexander Technique, which re-educates people in the use of their bodies, and helps them to acquire healthier and more relaxed physical habits.

When a complete cure is not possible the chiropractor will try to make it clear to the patient that the damaged or weakened area of the spine is liable to remain vulnerable, even though treatment has provided relief. Then it is up to the patient not to overdo physical activity or undertake tasks like heavy lifting which will make their problem worse. In such cases the chiropractor may suggest, after the initial course of treatments, that the patient should come in for 'maintenance' treatment every few months. He may also supply aids, such as support-belts for heavy activities; sometimes even a change of job may be advised.

A young nurse, Miss R., had a recurrent back problem, diagnosed by a doctor as a 'slipped disc'. 'The hospital physiotherapist did everything he could, but he said, "I'm not sure what I'm treating – it's not like a slipped disc." When I went to see a chiropractor he examined me and took X-rays, and told me I hadn't got a disc problem at all.' Her back troubles were caused by the fact that the spinous processes were missing from two of her vertebrae, weakening the spine. Her chiropractor gave her exercises to strengthen her back, but advised her that nursing, with the standing and lifting involved, was clearly not appropriate for her.

She took his advice and began re-training as a health visitor while working in a less strenuous private nursing post. 'As a nurse,' she says, 'my chiropractor has done me more good than any doctor. And he'll sit down and talk to you!'

CHAPTER THREE

JOINT PROBLEMS

AND SPORTS INJURIES

'The neck-bone's connected to the shoulder bone ...'

After the low back, the most common problem area –
affecting around 30 per cent of chiropractic patients – is the
neck. The cervical spine, composed of the vertebrae of the
neck, is quite a delicate structure which has to support the
skull, which weighs ten to fifteen pounds. As with backs,
stiff and painful necks tend to creep up on one over time,
and are often caused by bad posture or sitting for long
hours at work in a fixed position – drivers, typists and
VDU operators are particularly vulnerable. Habitual tension is another common cause: the neck and shoulders
easily tighten under stress, and in some people remain
tense, causing the muscles to tighten up around the joints
and decreasing the blood supply to the area.

Untreated, a joint fixation or subluxation in the neck can
lead to a variety of other aches and pains, as well as becoming increasingly painful and stiff in itself. Some neck
conditions relate to pelvic problems, causing or being
caused by them; although there is more than one school of
thought about this, if you consider the spine as a continuous flexible rod it makes sense that a change at one end
should bring about a change at the other. For example, a
man who presented himself at a chiropractic clinic with
low-back pain was surprised to be asked, after X-rays had
been taken, what had happened to his neck twenty years
earlier. On the X-ray no mechanical problem could be seen
in his lower back, but the results of an accident could be
seen in the neck.

In addition, an estimated 35 per cent of shoulder and arm pains originate in the neck through the mechanism of referred pain; headaches are another very common consequence. Manipulation of the neck can reverse this process, bringing all-round relief.

A forty-five-year-old woman, Mrs F., suffered continual severe arm pain for a year. The hospital she attended prescribed pain-killers without taking X-rays; the efforts of two osteopaths and two physiotherapists brought about no improvement. By the time she saw a chiropractor she was extremely worried that her pain might be due to cancer. The chiropractor's X-rays reassured her that there was no cancer, but there were joint restrictions at the base of her neck and in the mid thoracic area, causing the arm pain by trapping a nerve. After only four treatments Mrs F. was very much improved, and maintained the improvement by visiting the chiropractor for a check-up every two or three months.

Irritation of nerves in the neck can cause a number of aches and pains in the shoulders and arms, often quite severe. Conditions labelled 'neuritis', 'bursitis', 'neuralgia', 'rheumatism', 'frozen shoulder', 'fibrositis' and 'pins and needles' can all stem from nerves affected by joints in the neck; the neck can also be a contributory factor in tennis elbow, inflammation of the tendons at the elbow. Chiropractic adjustment can deal very effectively with these painful conditions, and exercises and awareness of posture will help maintain the benefits of treatment.

The idea of having the neck manipulated can be alarming to some people; good chiropractors are conscious of this, and encourage patients to relax beforehand. They do not twist the head forcefully, as some people fear, but may apply a gentle stretch or a rapid, light thrust (BCA and IPC adjustments will differ in this area particularly). In fact, although accidents have occurred in manipulating necks, they are very few and far between. In the Middle

East and India barbers often perform it on their customers as an extra service, with no ill-effects and indeed positive beneficial ones. 'You walk out into the heat feeling happier and taller!' remarks a doctor who has experienced this.

Joint Pains and Stress

Feeling better after having the neck manipulated is quite a common experience. Susan Moore tells me: 'People often say that with a neck problem they feel a bit depressed or lethargic, but once they've had the neck treated they suddenly feel as if a weight's been lifted off, the depression goes, and they feel a lot more lively. I don't think any good research has been done into why this happens, but all the nerves leading out of the brain are contained in the neck, so it seems logical that it could affect your personality. The early chiropractors said that if you adjusted the top of the neck you would affect the rest of the body, and to me that is still true.'

Whether depression is causing a particular neck problem or vice versa may not always be clear, but manipulation may be able to break a potential cycle of depression – or worse. Between the skull and the top of the neck is a floating bone, the atlas, on which the head rocks when one nods. Although the degree of movement is slight this bone is very important, for if anything prevents that movement, the rest of the neck is put under strain by having much more work to do. Some people call the atlas 'the rocker', which would account for the expression 'off your rocker', implying that the head is off balance. Very occasionally an accident causing pressure on the spinal cord in this area can cause emotional disturbances, which can be cured by correct manipulation. (One chiropractor tells me that he brought about an episode of depression in a patient by a neck adjustment; this should not alarm readers as such an event is rare, and the chiropractor was able to rectify it when the patient complained!)

Stress and anxiety in turn can produce physical problems. 'Anxiety has a posture,' says George Walker. 'An anxious person may walk around with shoulders raised and chin jutting forward, eventually getting a lot of fatigue pain in the muscles and a jamming-up of the joints.' Continued stress produces on-going pain, which may need more than physical adjustment for the patient to recover fully. Mrs D. developed neck and shoulder pains after the death of her husband, which had affected her deeply. After three or four months of pain she decided to see a chiropractor, and was lucky in finding one who was also a sympathetic counsellor. 'Not only did he treat my shoulder and neck, but he counselled me at the same time. He explained to me how I was getting the pain, and that I was really bringing it on myself. I don't think I've ever been to a doctor who explained things like that; it gave me great faith in him. He helped me to see that I had to stop looking back and start looking forward and build a new life – which I have done! He also showed me how to relax, and I now try not to get het up about anything.'

Neck Injuries

Chiropractors take extra care if there is any history of previous damage to the neck. In a chiropractic clinic I was shown the X-rays of a man who had fractured a cervical vertebra in an accident; because of his other injuries this had not been noticed while he was in hospital, and the vertebra had healed itself out of position, in such a way that it could not be palpated. If the chiropractor had been unaware of this, some forms of manipulation would have been fatal, I was told. (The extremely light McTimoney technique would not do any damage in such a case, but this is an example of the value of X-rays.)

Chiropractic can and often does speed the healing of whiplash injury, which occurs when an accident like a car crash causes the head to jerk back beyond its normal range of movement. Provided the spine is stable and surgery is not required, standard medical treatment is to supply the patient with a collar to support the neck and keep it immobile; unfortunately this can lead to stiffness and further pain. An orthopaedic surgeon tells me that patients are often wrongly instructed to wear collars full-time; provided the spine is stable, the neck muscles can support the neck during the day. Apart from being worn as a safeguard while driving, a collar is best worn at night when the relaxed muscles put a strain on the joints, causing pain on waking. Also, immobility may not be the best treatment. Some recent hospital tests suggest that if the neck is mobilized following a whiplash injury (that is, taken through gentle turning movements by a physiotherapist), recovery is speedier and there is less likelihood of the neck stiffening up. Chiropractors would agree; a number of whiplash injuries have been successfully dealt with by early treatment (although full recovery may still take time). Some victims of whiplash injuries visit chiropractors after suffering pain for years, and can still obtain relief, if not a total cure.

Mr D., a forty-two-year-old scientist, experienced a whiplash injury as a passenger in a minor car crash. He had already had a 'dodgy neck' for ten years, suffering stiffness and aches; a physiotherapist had told him that he had got early arthritis which he would 'have to live with' and had prescribed a collar, which he found unbearable and didn't wear. I met him shortly after he had begun treatment for the whiplash injury, and he told me: 'After the accident my GP, who's usually very good, just felt my shoulders a bit and prescribed some pain-killers; he didn't see any need for X-rays.

'I'm a research scientist; I don't claim to know much about the human body but I just feel there has to be more than conventional medicine is offering. I don't know whether what the chiropractor's doing is based on anything scientifically proven, but I'm giving it a try! I'd always thought heat helped pain, but he surprised me by telling me to put an ice-pack on my neck to get the inflammation down. He does various things: he manipulates my neck and uses some instruments, including ultrasound which relieves pain and inflammation. I came within a week of the accident, and after six treatments in two weeks he has certainly produced some relief. At the beginning I was very depressed because I could only sleep flat on my back; now I can turn over in bed without being woken by pain, and my neck feels freer.'

After any kind of accident a chiropractic check-up is to be recommended once the hospital has done all it can. A teenage girl had a bad fall at school which left her with head injuries, and unconscious. After four days in hospital she was discharged, with a surgical collar to wear. Over the next two years she had frequent attacks of fainting followed by fits, which were diagnosed as epilepsy. Further hospital tests, including X-rays, could find no positive cause; her condition deteriorated, and she had to leave school. Eventually her mother decided to try chiropractic. After examination and X-rays the chiropractor diagnosed restriction of the arteries in the neck as the cause of both fainting and fits. She began improving immediately after treatment and six months later was so much better that she was able to return to school and live a normal, active life.

Skilled manipulation can on occasion help – without curing – the severely disabled. Graham Heale, a BCA chiropractor, told me how his father developed paraplegia after breaking his neck. 'When his feeling started to return he had some strength in his right arm, but didn't recover the use of that hand; he had also lost his sense of smell. But he took part in the Paraplegic Olympic Games as an archer, with his right hand taped to the bow, and won a Gold

Medal. Some fifteen years after the original accident he fell from his wheelchair, banging his head, and suffered headaches and neck pain for a long time. He finally went to a chiropractor who manipulated his neck – which I thought was pretty brave! It helped him a lot; he recovered the use of his hand and was able to grip a bow. His neck pain and headaches got better – and his sense of smell returned. He went on to become disabled sports Personality of the Year.'

Rheumatoid Arthritis

This very painful disease which leads to distortion of the joints has two phases: an active phase, when the joints are inflamed, and a non-active phase. Manipulation of the joints during the active, inflammatory phase is generally contra-indicated. Once the disease is in a non-active phase, or has burned itself out, sufferers may well find chiropractic of help. By this stage, unfortunately, the joints may have been damaged and have altered in structure, and the possibilities may be limited; how much can be achieved structurally will depend on individual cases. But chiropractors can still help here in the relief of pain.

Madeleine Brzeski, a McTimoney chiropractor, tells me that several people have come to her on first developing the disease, when they are wondering what is wrong with them. In some cases she has been able to help by advising on diet and also by counselling. The onset of rheumatoid arthritis is often preceded by a shock or trauma of some kind, which may be physical or emotional, and counselling can be very helpful to some people.

Other Joint Problems

Many people suffer from unspecified aches and pains which, in the elderly, tend to be given the blanket label of 'arthritis' or 'neuralgia'. It is surprising how many of these conditions can be helped by the right kind of treatment. Chiropractors can treat all the joints of the body, including ankles, knees, elbows and wrists, and problems like frozen shoulder, tennis elbow, tendonitis and carpel tunnel syndrome. Even the skull, face and jaw can be gently manipulated; pains in this area can stem from tension, and also often from badly fitting dentures or dental work which has left a 'bad bite'. (Some IPC chiropractors are currently working on these problems in collaboration with a dentist.)

In older people a quite common condition is 'subscapular pain', a pain underneath the shoulder-blade; it can be due to muscle tension or to nerve pain resulting from problems in the ribs or the spine. It may also appear as pain in the gall bladder or heart muscle, and if the patient has breathing difficulties it may appear as chest pain. Chiropractors are trained to distinguish where the pain comes from, and to treat it accordingly.

Another common problem in the elderly is osteoarthritis of the hip joint. Unlike osteoarthritis of the spine, this condition goes through a stage of inflammation; this is temporary, but once arthritis has set in it gradually gets more painful and disabling. Hip joint replacement operations are now standard orthodox treatment, and are usually very successful; however, people can experience a good deal of discomfort and difficulty while they wait, sometimes years, for an operation. Chiropractic can alleviate the pain and stiffness during this time, by improving the function of the joints in the spine, pelvis and the affected hip. Many chiropractors believe that by maintaining much more mobility than would otherwise be the case the operation can at least be postponed and possibly avoided altogether. One tells me that arthritis in the hip can be caused by a bad positioning of the joints; if the pelvis, hips and leg bones are properly aligned early enough, she says, deterioration can be halted; others, however, are sceptical about this.

At the other end of the scale, too much mobility can cause damage, strain and sprains, and chiropractors quite often find themselves dealing with sports injuries.

Sports Injuries

Sporting activities can result in a vast number of possible injuries which chiropractors are equipped to deal with, from muscle strain to serious accidents; jogging alone can produce problems in the back, knees, ankles, feet and toes! The more common injuries are strains to the muscles, sprains to joints or ligaments, and damage to the intervertebral discs.

After an accident chiropractors will take X-rays or have them taken. As well as fractures, some conditions like a severely torn cartilage may require surgery, and the chiropractor will refer these for hospital treatment. For strains and sprains, chiropractic treatment is largely similar to that offered by physiotherapy, including icepacks, bandaging, advice on how long to rest and the prescription of graduated exercise. (Some chiropractors also use treatments such as ultrasound.)

Graham Heale, while treating the full range of musculoskeletal problems, specializes in sports injuries and is official chiropractor to the British Professional Karate Association. He told me: 'Chiropractors have an extra little thing we can give sports people, which is an assessment of the joint and manipulation to speed up recovery. GPs usually leave sprains to get better on their own, but that isn't quick enough for sports people. My interest is not to convince somebody that they need manipulation; if they have a muscle sprain I'll treat that and show them how to apply an icepack or heat, and when to start exercise again. But it's often the inadequately treated problems of the past which make people vulnerable to sprains and strains in the future. So after the first twenty-four hours, and before beginning a rehabilitation programme, we would ensure that the joint functions normally by using manipulative procedures and working on the tendon or muscle itself, just to make sure that everything is where it ought to be and does the movements we expect it to do. A common misconception with the medical profession is to see that nothing is broken, and assume nothing else is wrong. But if a joint is sprained you may well have damaged the muscles as well.'

A chiropractor is also likely to examine the whole body, not just the painful area. For example, a fall or rugby tackle heavy enough to displace a knee cartilage may also have knocked the pelvis out of position; if so, full recovery will require straightening the pelvis as well as treating the knee.

The very personal type of service provided by practitioners like Graham Heale includes observing people's techniques during their rehabilitation process – watching how they run, or grip a tennis racquet, for instance. One of his patients, David Bainsfair, a Bedfordshire Badminton League player, told me how he had been treated for 'the worst case of tennis elbow Graham had ever seen!

'It was so bad I was thinking of packing up the game – it was too painful even to use the telephone! My doctor gave me cortisone injections and seemed to think the only answer was to stop playing. Then at the local hospital I was given ultrasound, which didn't help. After six months, someone suggested that chiropractic might do something for me, so I went along. Graham was my last hope really – I do love the game! When he examined me he reckoned he would get it better by Christmas. He found I had a weak spot on the right side of my neck, probably caused through doing a lot of driving in my work. He worked on that first, and told me to use cold compresses for my arm to reduce the inflammation – I'd much rather have that than anti-inflammatory drugs. He gave me some exercises to do, very light at first, such as squeezing a ball. After two or three months of this and regular treatment, mainly to my arm once he'd fixed my neck, I started being able to use the telephone.

'What also helped was that Graham found the *cause* of the problem. He asked me to take my racquet along, and it turned out the handle was too small, so that over the years my wrist and arm action with too tight a grip had caused wear and tear on the elbow. I bought a lighter racquet and bandaged up the handle to give me more grip. By Christmas I did start playing again, though at first I had to resort to a backhand serve. One of my colleagues is a badminton coach, and I went and talked to the youngsters he was coaching about the importance of getting the right racquet grip!

'I wish more people with tennis elbow knew about chiropractic. The attention I got was fantastic. The hospital never suggested I could do anything for myself. I still carry on with the exercises every morning, and it's good knowing I can help myself.'

Chiropractors are particularly interested in prevention; many of the aches, pains and back problems that arise in running or cycling, for example, are not caused by the activities themselves, but by being unfit to start with. 'You shouldn't do a sport to get fit, you should get fit to do the sport!' Graham says. Having an expert check your style, too, can prevent future mishaps. A faulty running style, for instance, can cause injuries if shoulders are too tense; the roll of the hips can affect the knees, ankles and feet, while splay feet can injure the knee joint.

While it's obviously an advantage for sports people to go to someone with a special interest, most chiropractors regularly treat sports injuries – some of them not immediately obvious. Martin Cooper at the age of twenty-six is an amateur triathlete (which involves swimming, cycling and running). As a result of a motor-cycle accident some years before, he had a back problem. 'Every now and again it would "go" and I'd find myself on the floor, literally unable to move. Then it would suddenly get better again, after three or four days. I'd been to a number of doctors; none of them even asked me to take my shirt off, and they told me there was nothing wrong with me. Eventually, when my back was quite bad, I went to see a McTimoney chiropractor, and since having a course of treatments I no longer get twinges or pain.

'But most important for me, it got rid of another problem that I thought was separate from my back, which was that I had terrible stomach upsets when I was running.' (Stomach cramps and diarrhoea are fairly common among runners.) 'I'd been to doctors and had a barium meal X-ray and was again told that nothing was wrong, and I was quite prepared to believe that – I thought it was something everyone got. The chiropractor explained that the nerves in the area of my back problem were affecting my stomach and fixed both at the same time. It was marvellous – manna from heaven!'

Which leads us neatly to the subject of the less obvious problems with which chiropractic can sometimes be surprisingly successful.

CHAPTER FOUR

WHAT ELSE CAN

CHIROPRACTORS TREAT?

The early chiropractors – and some recent ones – antagonized doctors by claiming that chiropractic could cure all kinds of diseases. Unfortunately this over-enthusiasm has led the medical profession to discount those beneficial side-effects that *do* occur. Yet conditions like migraine, vertigo, bronchial asthma, catarrh, indigestion, constipation and menstrual disorders are relieved often enough for it to be more than coincidence. And most experienced chiropractors will have experienced at least one case where deafness or poor vision has been improved. (Similar effects are familiar to practitioners of other forms of manipulation, like osteopaths.)

Probably a fairly typical picture of the type and proportion of such cases is that extracted from the questionnaires returned by patients to the McTimoney Chiropractic School in 1983, the first 2,480 of which have been analysed. Sixty-nine patients reported relief of migraine and headaches; other problems relieved were stomach and digestive problems (25 patients), followed by asthma and bronchial complaints (18), menstrual problems (17), kidneys (13) and hay fever (10). Benefits to the senses (i.e. eyesight, hearing, balance, and relief of tinnitus) totalled 17, while smaller numbers were helped with haemorrhoids (1), eczema (3), anaemia (1) and car sickness (1).

The New Zealand Commission designated this kind of cure 'Type O' (organic conditions), in contrast with 'Type M' (musculo-skeletal disorders). Although Type O cures only constituted 7 per cent of the disorders reported to the

Commission, the rest being Type M, the 7 per cent consisted of ninety-nine ailments which patients said had responded to chiropractic treatment. While pointing out that some alleged cures may have been examples of self-remission or the side-effects of treatment for something else, the Commission concluded that some cases 'seem hard to explain on any basis other than that the treatment given by the chiropractor brought about the cure'.

Among the witnesses testifying to the Commission was an experienced medical practitioner, described as 'highly intelligent and open-minded', who 'took the view that his patients were entitled to the treatment which was most appropriate for their condition – including treatment by a chiropractor – as long as it was safe for the particular patient ... He had seen for himself what he believed to be the benefits of chiropractic treatment both to his own family and to his patients ... He told the Commission of some remarkable cases in which he believed that chiropractic treatment had successfully cured, or significantly relieved, asthma, deafness, narcolepsy (a condition characterized by sudden attacks of an uncontrollable desire to sleep), chorea (St Vitus dance) and eczema. He asserted the effectiveness of chiropractic treatment in some cases of diabetes, not as a cure, but as a means of enabling certain patients significantly to lower their insulin intake.'

How Do These Cures Occur?

There seem to be two processes at work here. One is the phenomenon of referred pain: it is medically recognized that aches and pains in the head, chest and abdomen can stem from the spine. According to Dr John Paterson, 30 per cent of all headaches are vertebral in origin, and so is a good deal of chest and abdominal pain. As he somewhat idiosyncratically puts it, 'If you turn the patient over, in quite a high proportion of cases abnormal physical signs will be found *if they are sought* ... The honest cardiologist will admit that with 20 per cent of the chaps he checks out he draws a blank.'

So it seems feasible that the heart patient whom Palmer 'cured' had been misdiagnosed. Apparent angina or heart pains may be referred pain from the spine, which adjustment can relieve. Strictly speaking these are not Type O complaints, although until a patient receives relief through chiropractic their doctor may be treating them as such.

However, chiropractic does sometimes relieve genuine Type O conditions, a more mysterious process. The hypothesis is that this comes about through the activity of the nervous system; there certainly seems no other explanation for it. As we have seen, the central nervous system branches out from the spine to link up with different parts of the body and with the autonomic nervous system, which controls the digestive system, including the liver, pancreas and bowel, kidney function, and so on. It can be imagined as a vast telephone network, and the theory is that a spinal subluxation can cause a jamming in communications, preventing an organ from functioning fully. Adjusting the relevant vertebra restores the flow of nervous impulses to that organ, allowing it to resume normal function. Another more generalized explanation is that manipulating the spine 'normalizes' the activity of the central nervous system, thereby improving the functioning of the whole body; thus symptoms not directly connected with the spine clear up as a result of an over-all boost in health.

Dr Goodheart, the founder of Applied Kinesiology, has found a connection with the acupuncture meridians, each of which has an associated point in the spine which would also be affected by adjustment; the action still occurs through the nervous system but takes, as it were, a different route. 'For example, the nerve supply to the stomach comes off the spine at a point between the shoulder blades,

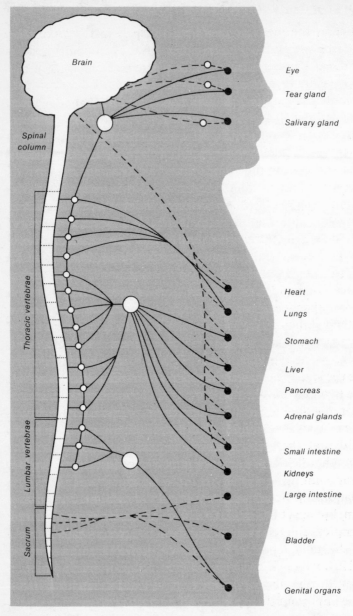

How the spinal cord relates to the rest of the body: the nerve connections leading from the brain to the vital organs

whereas the meridian system comes off just below where the ribs end. It doesn't fit neurologically, but when you fix it there the person's stomach function remarkably improves,' he says. Many chiropractors would agree with Dr Goodheart that chiropractic is not valued highly enough for its potential effects on the nervous system.

As a lay person, I can quite easily believe that my spine is linked via my nervous system to non-bony bits of me, and that stimulating the nervous system by adjusting vertebrae can stimulate healing elsewhere, just as in acupuncture stimulating a point on the foot can boost liver function. However, to scientifically trained minds this may sound like nonsense. Although chiropractors tell me that neurophysiologists find the hypothesis worth entertaining, most doctors and orthopaedic surgeons will dismiss Type O cures as coincidence, or the result of the placebo effect – the power of suggestion on the patient.

One difficulty that medicine has with the concept of Type O cures is that it has so divided the human body that there is one type of specialist for the stomach and another for the spine, and never the twain shall meet; links between the two may never be seen. Another is that it has not so far been possible to demonstrate *scientifically* how these cures work. Alan Breen, Research Director at the AECC, says, 'Although there is more research in this field than possibly any other field in chiropractic, results have so far been very disappointing – almost a damp squib. There definitely is a relationship between spinal function and the nervous system, but apart from the fact that the neurology is very, very complex, the relationship is just not predictable enough to be clinically dependable.'

However, if Type O cures have not yet been scientifically proved, they have not been scientifically *disproved* either. The important thing, as *Chiropractic in New Zealand* states, 'is whether a particular form of treatment has *in fact* achieved a particular result ... The main point, in human terms, is that the chiropractors in some cases appeared to succeed in relieving great suffering and hardship where more orthodox methods had apparently failed.'

Lack of Predictability

The problem with Type O cures is that they *are* unpredictable and often unexpected: an elderly lady visits a chiropractor for her arthritis and finds her hearing improved; someone else comes in with pains in the upper back, and mentions in passing, after treatment, that their indigestion has cleared up. Few patients go to chiropractors specifically for this sort of problem, though once a practitioner acquires a reputation for 'being good with' migraines or deafness he may well attract similar cases. But he can only try to treat them if there is a spinal subluxation directly relating to the organ concerned, and even then cannot predict the outcome. 'We don't treat headaches,' says one. 'We treat people with headaches for subluxations.'

There are some problems like migraine and asthma for which chiropractic might be worth trying more often than it is – on the understanding that no reputable chiropractor will guarantee a cure. The cases described below are examples of what can happen, but it should be stressed that they are what researchers refer to as 'anecdotal': stories reported by patients, but not based on scientifically controlled studies.

Headaches and Migraine

Chiropractic can be very effective in alleviating headaches and migraine: in fact the New Zealand Commission classified such cures as Type M rather than Type O, since when they occur there seems to be a clear relationship with problems of the cervical spine.

Tension headaches, caused by stress or overwork, are caused by muscle contractions in the neck, particularly at the base of the skull, the effects of which spread into the head. They differ from the full-blown migraine, which can include temporary partial loss of vision or the impression of flashing lights, and vomiting, and occur regularly in those unfortunate enough to suffer from them. Migraines (of which there is more than one type) may be hereditary, and can be triggered by foods such as cheese, chocolate and wine. They are preceded by a constriction of the blood vessels to the head, which causes the visual disturbances; the blood vessels then dilate, producing the headache. In some cases the cause can be traced to a disturbance of the spine affecting that part of the nervous system which controls the blood vessels.

Chiropractic treatment consists of adjusting the part of the spine which is causing the disturbance. The exact adjustments will depend on which type of headache is involved, and can also vary from patient to patient; generally a course of treatments is needed.

In the questionnaires completed by McTimoney patients, 30 gave migraine as their reason for visiting a chiropractor; 29 of these reported improvement, 24 by over 60 per cent. Forty others who visited practitioners with other muscular complaints reported relief from migraine as a bonus, 17 had complete relief and the others some relief. In addition, there were some 78 cases of cured headaches, or of considerable improvement. The patients included people like Anna, a hospital technician, who visited a chiropractor for painful sciatica in her legs – and found that not only was that relieved, but her migraines stopped too.

Headaches may be accompanied by vertigo. A lady of seventy visited a BCA chiropractor after two years of frequent headaches accompanied by attacks of dizziness and nausea, which had begun shortly after she had been under stress looking after her sick father. She had several of these unpleasant attacks a week, lasting for two hours at a time. Her GP prescribed drugs which helped once an attack had started, but didn't prevent them. The chiropractor's orthopaedic and neurological tests proved negative, and an X-ray of her cervical spine showed mild degenerative changes. On palpation, fixations were found in the upper cervical joints, and the chiropractor gave specific manipulative therapy to this area of the neck. The patient had five treatments in a month, during which she had only one fairly mild attack. After that she was advised to come back for a check-up every three months. This kind of relief must make all the difference to a person's life.

Other Problems Connected with the Head

Sinus problems can respond well to gentle manipulation of the head and face, and so occasionally can on-going pain following dental treatment.

Occasionally eyesight can improve. Alison Gordon-Creed started suffering eye-strain while studying in the evenings with the McTimoney School. Out of curiosity she had her eyes tested by three different opticians, all of whom agreed she needed glasses, though each made out a different prescription! Having had no chiropractic treatment for some time, she decided to see whether further treatment would help. After four sessions with her chiropractor she was tested again by one of the opticians, and to her delight her vision was pronounced 20-20. However, she herself had no success with a woman patient whose eyesight had deteriorated during pregnancy. 'We agreed to try three treatments experimentally,' she told me, 'and in the event I gave her five, but her eyes didn't improve. There can be so many causes; I thought she might be suffering from a vitamin deficiency, so I referred her to a naturopath.'

There has been more than one case of relief of mental problems resulting from an accident. *Chiropractic in New Zealand* tells the story of a bright, intelligent schoolgirl who had cranial surgery to remove a blood clot following an accident at the age of eleven. Her memory was badly affected and she found herself at the bottom of her class, while at home her behaviour became difficult. On leaving school she found employment doing simple repetitive work for an understanding employer, but was frustrated by her inability to concentrate or remember things; she could not go on a simple journey without taking notes reminding her which bus or train to catch. After consulting several unorthodox practitioners without success, she visited a chiropractor. He found an obvious subluxation which he adjusted straight away. Later she phoned her mother, crying with joy, because she had found her way home from the chiropractor's without using notes. After one slight relapse she continued to improve: she began playing the piano and reading, and travelled overseas by herself. Her mother commented: 'I have got back the daughter I lost.'

Hearing Problems

A BCA chiropractor says: 'If I set out to specialize in treating deafness, I wouldn't make a very good living!' Nevertheless, some cases do respond, and when they do they must resemble D. D. Palmer's cure of Harvey Lillard's deafness, in that the deafness related to a particular spinal subluxation.

'Rarely is deafness a primary problem for people who come looking for help,' says Steve Carpenter, 'but very often one can rid elderly people of the need to use hearing aids. My own thesis is that there's an area in the neck that is strongly related to the ear. I never claim to cure deafness, but if there is a mechanical problem there I tell the patient that I shall be treating the whole of their spine, and to let me know if they notice improvements in their hearing. It is remarkable how many people say their hearing has improved. With tinnitus I get mixed results, with an improvement rate of about 50 per cent – why, I don't know.'

Alison Gordon-Creed found herself getting requests to treat deafness after helping one woman who had been deaf in her left ear all her life. 'It's early days yet,' she told me. 'You certainly get some change, but there's no way you can give one adjustment and they walk out able to hear. There are two or three specific places I would treat in the thoracic and cervical spine – the second cervical vertebra affects the nerve supply to the middle ear. But it is often the effect of the pelvis, the way they sit and what the muscles and bones are doing there, that makes the second cervical vertebra go out of place all the time. So there's no point in just adjusting the vertebra; you have to correct what's causing it, and that is quite hard. It's sometimes tied up with years of bad posture.'

Asthma, Bronchial Complaints and Allergy

Asthma and other breathing problems can often be helped, though manipulation seems to be less effective in asthmatic adults than in children, probably because of the law of fixation. Even so, some adults do gain relief. A man in his seventies visited a chiropractor after injuring his head in an accident; after treatment, not only was his head better but he had lost his asthma. The asthma recurred from time to time, but could always be relieved by a chiropractic adjustment.

Treating breathing problems usually involves adjustment to the neck and may include the rib area. Chris

Pearcey, a McTimoney chiropractor, was visited by a woman with chest pains resulting from the strain of emphysema, an unpleasant disease which restricts breathing. 'There is no way I could treat the emphysema,' he says, 'but I was able to relieve her of pain in her ribs and diaphragm caused by the stress of difficult breathing.'

With asthma there is an allergy factor, of course; other allergic symptoms like eczema are sometimes treated successfully. If something is triggered by an allergy, how can manipulation affect it? Dr Arne Christensen, Dean of the AECC, explains: 'A lot of us are allergic to various substances, but within a normal band. But if there is then a biomechanical disturbance we start to react outside our normal physiology. Because we call it asthma, we shouldn't be blinded to the fact that other things may be playing a part. If the biomechanical problem is the *cause* of the asthmatic problem, in children it can clear up very quickly. The hypothesis is that if there is interference with the nervous system, you may lose control over other physiological functions.'

Steve Carpenter recently cured a patient of both eczema and migraines, by manipulation alone. 'Nobody knows the causes for eczema but it is worse under stress,' he says. 'Why can't a body cope with a certain compound? Is it the fact that the nervous system is not working correctly? So my approach to allergy is to make sure that the spine is working well enough for long enough to get rid of the mechanical aspects. One patient of mine went to an allergy-testing clinic for a check-up with regard to sinus trouble; she was pronounced allergic to almost every compound you cound find, with less than 10 per cent that she wasn't allergic to. Yet she is relatively healthy! I don't believe that the body is as allergic to things as is made out, and if it is, then the nervous system is responsible.'

Some chiropractors may prescribe a change in diet as well. Stan Harding says: 'If the body becomes very toxic due to years of wrong eating habits, I try to encourage the patient to eat a more healthy diet which will gradually clean the body out, lowering the level of toxicity; the allergies will then often disappear. Acquiring allergies through a slow toxic build-up in the body can be compared with allowing a tap to drip into a sink: it can go on for years with no apparent harm and then suddenly the sink overflows. If we lower the level of the water and stop further drips, the problem is solved.'

Abdominal Pains and Digestive Problems

Abdominal pain, like chest pain, is sometimes misdiagnosed referred pain coming from the back. 'How many surgeons take out a perfectly normal appendix every now and again?' wonders Dr Paterson. And Susan Moore says: 'Very often a patient will complain of indigestion going right through to their back. No amount of Rennies or Alka-Seltzer is going to make them better if it's a spinal adjustment they need.'

Conversely, some back pains do come from unhealthy organs. It is part of the chiropractor's skill to find out which is causing what. For example, you might have a pain caused by a subluxation in the upper back, an area that relates to the liver. Has the liver caused the subluxed vertebra, or is the subluxation affecting your liver? By the time you reach a chiropractor a kind of circuit may have been set up in which each keeps triggering the other. As James Rousseau explained to me: 'Where you have, say, an impinged nerve in the thoracic spine, due to injury or faulty posture, there is then a reflex from the spine to the liver, called a somato-visceral response. But if you have damaged the organ, this can show itself as back pain; this is a viscero-somatal reflex. In both cases there may well be a subluxation in the part of the spine connecting with the area, which can be relieved by manipulation. However, if the problem starts with faulty nutrition the back pain will recur.

'Overtaxing the liver by excessive drugs, alcohol or coffee, for example, can produce pain between the shoulder blades. If that isn't corrected it will come back and keep firing the nerves, and the muscles can go into spasm. The spasm in turn starts interfering with the nerve supply to the liver. An adjustment breaks that cycle by easing the muscle spasm and stimulating the nerve to the organ, hopefully getting a flow of energy to it. But if the problem is, say, excessive coffee-drinking, you can go on adjusting till the cows come home. You will maybe make the person feel a little more comfortable, but if he goes home and continues to overtax the liver, two weeks later he'll return with back pain. Then you have to ask, "What's going on here?"'

Genuine digestive problems like constipation, diarrhoea and diverticulitis have been known to clear up through chiropractic treatment (as we saw in the last chapter). But again, as Susan Moore says, 'It depends on the cause. Is it a spastic colon, or diverticulitis, or is the back irritating the nerve supply to the bowel? Constipation, for instance, can clear up just through treating the back, but not every time. If patients have that problem I might suggest changing their diet – though you have to get to know people before you make radical changes in their lifestyle! But sometimes constipation can lead to lower-back pain, and both can be altered by diet.

'A patient of mine in her early twenties had back trouble; she saw various specialists, had physiotherapy and what have you, but didn't make any progress. The physio sent her to me because he thought some proper manipulation might help, rather than just mobilization. After a couple of treatments it became apparent that her back pain was related to constipation. She'd already been told she had bowel problems and should have a high fibre diet. I got her to write down what she ate for two weeks and found that although she *thought* she was eating a high fibre diet it consisted of foods that are actually very low in fibre. So we changed her diet and within about a month she was regular and the back had settled down remarkably.'

Hiatus hernia is another digestive problem, but of a mechanical nature. A hernia in the diaphragm at the point where the oesophagus goes through it to the stomach can cause acid regurgitation, and a good deal of pain and discomfort. Some cases may require surgery, but the chiropractor can often treat it effectively with a combination of spinal adjustment and assisted breathing.

Diabetes

No chiropractor would claim to cure diabetes, but diabetic patients being treated for other problems often find their need for insulin drastically reduced, presumably because the nerve supply to the pancreas has been improved. (Similar effects have been noted in diabetics practising both autogenic relaxation and yoga.) So it is obviously important for a diabetic patient visiting a chiropractor to have their insulin requirements regularly checked. Diabetics often breathe poorly, too; chiropractors can help here by releasing tight muscles in the ribs and diaphragm, and recommending breathing exercises.

Kidney Problems and High Blood Pressure

High blood pressure can relate to poorly functioning kidneys, which in turn often relate to back pain. It is quite common for blood pressure to be lower after treatment; kidney problems such as water-retention (oedema) can respond, too. A defect of medical treatment in this area is that the drugs which are prescribed for blood pressure (as well as for other conditions like arthritis) add an extra burden to the kidneys which have to eliminate the chemicals from the body. Chiropractors obviously have to work carefully here; they cannot advise patients to give up medically prescribed drugs, but treatment may lessen the need for them. Clearly, the ideal solution if possible is for the chiropractor to work in cooperation and communication with the doctor.

A New Zealand patient, Mrs M., visited a chiropractor for a whiplash injury, for which he treated her quickly and successfully. She also suffered from high blood pressure, water retention and headaches, and he told her that her blood pressure could be expected to go down and that her water retention problem would also improve. Although she was confident in his ability to treat her neck, she was doubtful about the other conditions. But, as she told the New Zealand Commission, 'To my surprise, and great satisfaction, everything that he has told me has eventuated. My blood pressure is now normal (I take no blood pressure tablets) and my water retention has improved about 75 per cent (I now take tablets about once weekly instead of every day).' She was sensible enough to have these conditions monitored by her doctor, who was, not unnaturally, surprised when her blood pressure reverted to normal. (The Commission was allowed to see her medical records for confirmation.)

Relief from water retention can be quite dramatic. The receptionist of a BCA chiropractor suffered from bladder problems and came into work one morning complaining that she'd stopped passing water. The chiropractor asked her to bring in a sample next day, but meanwhile gave her low back an emergency treatment in the lunch-hour. She spent the afternoon rushing to the loo!

Stress

A number of patients have commented on an over-all feeling of well-being and greater energy after treatment. I have already touched on the subject of emotional stress, which can cause mechanical problems in the neck, shoulders, arms and lower back. Pain in turn creates further stress, and its removal can break this negative cycle, bringing about real emotional relief and improved general health.

Sometimes stress has far-reaching effects. I have found it difficult to decide how to classify the following story. Does it come under neck problems? Heart trouble? Addiction? Or just stress-ridden modern man?

Peter is now thirty-four; his problems probably originated with a number of accidents when he was young, including the loss of an eye. In his mid twenties he developed a 'nervous stomach' for which his doctor prescribed Valium, and for the next five years he took 30–40mg a day; it was not yet recognized that tranquillizers are highly addictive and should not be taken for more than four or five months at a time, nor that they can actually produce the anxiety they are supposed to relieve. After five years Peter began to suffer from dizziness and severe headaches. Several doctors told him it was 'nerves' and prescribed more Valium. Six months later, on 60mg of Valium a day, he was found to have heart trouble, with palpitations, disorientation, and severe neck and back pains. Valium is a muscle relaxant and Peter is convinced that it caused his heart rate to slow down. He was given a pacemaker which set his heart rate and for a short time was well except for the back tension, which spread to his chest; further medication didn't help.

Meanwhile, worried about his high Valium intake, Peter cut it down to 10mg a day, unaware that cutting down can produce very unpleasant withdrawal symptoms, including panic attacks. His tension grew worse and he began to lose the use of his arms. A psychiatrist told him he was low in confidence and doubted his own health – which was true, but Peter knew his pain was real, not in his mind. He waited three months to see a neurosurgeon, who said there was nothing wrong with his central nervous system, and refused to consider Peter's suggestion that the Valium might have affected his nerves. Peter felt for a while as if he were going mad (a common experience among tranquillizer addicts); he withdrew into a shell, unable to sleep, eat or go out.

Then he met a friend who had formerly been on tranquillizers but who now looked extremely well. He told Peter he had been to see McTimoney chiropractor Chris Pearcey. With nothing to lose, Peter decided to visit him. He not only got a sympathetic hearing, but received the first effective treatment for his problems. Chris found that his atlas was quite severely out of line, most of the vertebrae of the neck and upper back were subluxated, and his pelvis was out of true. It is quite possible that this originally started with the loss of his eye putting a strain on Peter's neck, since he had to turn his head further than normal to look to one side; the neck problems in turn could well have led to the nervous symptoms for which he was originally prescribed Valium.

Peter was still slowly cutting down and suffering withdrawal symptoms; here Chris helped by recommending him to come off stimulants like tea and coffee (and Peter helped himself by complying) while relieving the physical tensions caused by drug withdrawal. After a few months of regular treatment, starting weekly and extending to six-weekly, Peter's neck, spine and pelvis problems were sorted out, and he was able to cut out Valium completely. A recent pacemaker check showed that his heart rhythm had returned to normal – which seems to validate his theory about the effects of Valium. He describes himself as 're-born'.

There are all kinds of reasons for stress. Like back pain, it is a modern plague. The public and the medical profession are beginning to realize that chemical suppression is not the answer. While all kinds of factors may be involved, stress is rarely 'all in the mind'; it affects the body in very tangible ways, producing muscle spasm and spinal subluxations which need physical treatment. In Peter's case mental stress seems to have resulted from biomechanical factors, rather than the other way round. Early chiropractic treatment could have prevented him from having to endure years of increasing mental pain. As it is, he was fortunate to find a therapist who not only offered him time and compassion and took his problems seriously, but the physical skills to treat his physical symptoms.

CHAPTER FIVE

CHIROPRACTIC

FOR WOMEN

Women have specific problems which can be greatly helped by chiropractic. Whether they are mothers, nurses, dentists, hairdressers – or chiropractors – their lives involve a lot of standing, bending and heavy lifting, all of which can lead to back strain or worse. The working conditions of the secretary, typist and VDU operator are often far from ideal; they tend to sit for long hours with their heads turned in one direction, often at keyboards which are too high, on chairs the wrong height for the working surface, and it's not surprising that they often suffer from neck and shoulder tension leading to headaches and eye-strain. Women's work is not restricted to offices, of course; many, like nurses and farmers' wives, have to do a lot of lifting, while for mothers the physical burdens of pregnancy and child care can place major strains on the back.

Susan Moore, a thirty-two-year-old BCA chiropractor, treats both sexes but inevitably attracts a lot of women patients. 'Many women prefer to see a woman, particularly if they're middle-aged and have a lot of flab! They sometimes think a woman is more understanding, as well,' she told me. This may in some cases be true, although most women patients report very favourably on the respect and care with which they are treated by chiropractors of either sex. However, the BCA is somewhat male-dominated (although this is changing, about two-thirds of its members in 1986 are men), and a male chiropractor has commented that there is a danger of falling into the trap of chauvinism. Susan's male colleagues originally found it difficult to accept a woman in their practice, fearing that men would find it embarrassing to be treated by a woman. However, she found that once male patients realized that she was a professional with a professional attitude, their embarrassment disappeared and Susan now has a well-established practice.

The majority of women patients come with lower-back pain. Susan Moore's female patients have included members of a women's group who have suffered injuries through sport or work – one was a painter and decorator and one a heavy goods vehicle driver. She sees a number of mothers with young children, who get back trouble from the combination of lifting toddlers, gardening and housework. (Turning mattresses, according to an American practitioner, is about the worst thing you can do for the health of your back!) Nurses are frequent visitors to chiropractic clinics; at one I visited, three nurses or ex-nurses were being treated in one morning.

During the diagnostic session chiropractors take into account that some lower-back pains may arise from internal disorders rather than from the spine itself; in women these can be gynaecological problems, such as fibroids or pelvic infection caused by IUDs. Conversely, a medical expert informs me that hysterectomies are sometimes carried out needlessly, when pain from the spine is referred to the pelvis; in such cases, if the medical diagnosis is in any doubt, a check-up with a chiropractor may show that an operation is unnecessary. Kidney problems and constipation can also cause back pains; gall-bladder trouble, to which women are particularly prone, can create pain in many other parts of the body. So the chiropractor will first check whether there is a genuine back problem, and if there isn't will suggest that the patient returns to her doctor for a further check-up.

'Doctors often say it's a back problem without doing a full examination,' says Susan. 'It's actually quite difficult to tell whether it's the back or something else, but a chiropractor can detect if there's a definite back problem there. If I can find nothing wrong with the back I'll ask about the patient's periods, whether she's got an IUD, or suffers from nausea, and so on.'

Having lower-back problems treated is not only a relief in itself; there may be bonuses. Since there is both a muscular and a nervous link between the uterus and a section of the spine, adjustment can lead to easier menstruation, with periods becoming more regular and less painful. Occasionally women report having early, late or extra heavy periods after the first treatment, but after this their periods should normalize.

Pre-menstrual tension and menopausal symptoms are less likely to be affected, since they involve the complexities of the hormonal system; however, the relief of stress resulting from treatment may help by reducing over-all tension. The chiropractor may also give basic dietary advice, such as cutting down on salt and coffee, but if symptoms are serious he or she may refer patients to an expert. Susan often sends pre-menstrual sufferers to a homoeopath whom she knows to be successful with this all-too-common problem.

Many women are troubled – and indeed worried – by back pain following a gynaecological operation like a hysterectomy or D&C. This may simply be due to the way in which these operations are performed, which puts a lot of strain on the lower back, so chiropractic treatment may well relieve it. (If a woman with back problems has to have this kind of operation, she should tell the surgeon beforehand; he will usually arrange for her back to be supported by pillows during the operation.)

Pregnancy and Birth

Among Susan Moore's patients are many women who

would like to become pregnant, but wonder if their backs can stand it. 'I always say that if you've got a bad back, get that sorted out first and then get pregnant,' she says. 'I try to get them really fit, see them through the pregnancy, and check them after the birth. I also advise women on the pill to wait six months after coming off it before getting pregnant. Although many women don't get pregnant immediately after stopping the pill, some are pregnant within a month. There is a chance that these mothers will be lacking in certain vitamins and minerals of which the pill is known to deplete the body, and so I recommend waiting.'

No chiropractor would claim to treat sub-fertility but there have been occasional instances of a sub-fertile woman apparently being helped by chiropractic treatment, particularly when no obvious cause has been found for the condition. One fairly dramatic case was reported to the New Zealand Commission by the husband of a woman who had been unable to conceive during six years of marriage. The couple had been through intensive physical and gynaecological tests which could find no cause, and they eventually adopted two children. Then a friend persuaded the wife to consult a chiropractor, which she did without any expectations. The chiropractor found what the husband described as a 'misplaced vertebra', which he corrected in one treatment, and shortly afterwards she became pregnant. Unfortunately, such cases are very rare.

By contrast, all chiropractors would agree on the benefits of treatment during pregnancy. Carrying extra weight around while pregnant is a well-known cause of back pain, as is childbirth itself. It has sometimes been suggested that manipulation may be dangerous for pregnant women; this really seems to be far from true, although some manipulators might hesitate to treat a woman with a history of miscarriage, lest the treatment be blamed for a further episode. (One chiropractor would like the opportunity to check the pelvises of women who have had miscarriages, to see whether these might be caused by a spinal problem which adjustment could rectify.) In fact, for most women treatment offers both relief from back-ache before a birth and a spine in better shape after it.

A problem some chiropractors will treat in pregnancy is a narrow birth canal caused by an over-curved coccyx. Not all of them would undertake this unless the coccyx has actually been damaged, as it usually involves internal manipulation which is not very pleasant for either the patient or the practitioner; however, it can be done, and has been.

Current research indicates that babies while still in the womb are sensitive to and aware of noises around them, especially the sound of the human voice. Stan Harding encourages mothers to talk to their unborn babies, and his respect for the foetus is such that he will ask the baby's permission before treating a pregnant woman. 'I tell the mum I'm asking the baby; I put my hands on them and mentally ask, "Is it O K to treat you?", and if I get any strong negative feelings I don't treat. But that doesn't usually happen.'

Though obstetrics used to be taught in American chiropractic colleges, childbirth itself is not the province of chiropractors and they don't generally make dogmatic recommendations in the arguments for and against natural childbirth. Although squatting during the birth seems preferable for women who already have back trouble, each woman should be free to choose the position most comfortable for her. Chiropractors would, however, advise against having epidurals or other injections in the spine if these can be avoided; they may cause back pain later on.

Most women who have been through pregnancies first without and then with chiropractic treatment comment that the birth itself is easier after treatment. But one patient of Susan Moore's, a young nurse, had a traumatic birth following a thrombosis which kept her in bed for the last three months on blood-thinning drugs, which presumably also thinned the baby's blood. The baby became stuck in the birth canal, which was very painful for the mother's back. 'A couple of days after the birth,' Susan recalls, 'her doctor got so fed up with her asking to see her chiropractor that he rang up and asked me to please come and do a house call! I think he wanted anything for a quiet life. When I went I couldn't believe how dreadful the hospital beds were, all saggy in the middle with absolutely no support for the spine.' The mother is now doing fine, and is back at work part-time.

The female body prepares for birth by releasing a hormone called relaxin, which softens the ligaments so that they can stretch more easily for the birth. The drawback is that it also makes it much easier for the new mother to 'put her back out', just at a time when she is doing an extra amount of lifting, carrying and bending. So chiropractic treatment is to be recommended after the birth; babies can grow remarkably heavy very quickly, and back pain can worsen if left untreated. The chiropractor will also advise on back-strengthening exercises, and help the new mother to acquire habits that will prevent further trouble. For example, women commonly carry babies on their hip, very often on the same hip; changing sides from time to time will help to keep the muscles of the back working evenly.

Women's Work

Helping the patient to help herself is an important aspect of chiropractic. Chiropractors treat a good many office workers, and as well as suggesting preventative exercises they will discuss working arrangements and try to help optimize these. For example, typewriter or word-processor keys should be below elbow level, so that the operator does not have to hunch her shoulders; chairs should be low enough to sit with both feet flat on the ground, keeping the spine centred and straight, and these days document holders can be bought so that the copy-typist doesn't have to strain her neck by keeping her head tilted down and to one side. If bosses don't want the expense of buying really good typists' chairs, lumbar problems can still be eased or avoided by buying a triangular-shaped wedge to place on the chair seat; this helps to keep the spine straight by dropping the thighs downwards slightly.

Women who spend long hours at keyboards are also encouraged to stop every twenty minutes or so, so that their shoulders and necks don't become fixed. Taking a break to hunch and relax the shoulders and do a few gentle head-and-neck rolls can prevent strain.

Although patients may feel fully recovered after a series of treatments, once back trouble has occurred there may unfortunately be a permanent weakness there, so it is important for patients to follow their chiropractor's advice and look after themselves afterwards. The nurse whom Susan Moore treated for back pain after giving birth originally came for severe lower-back and leg pain, following heavy lifting at work and a low-back strain two years before. She responded to treatment very quickly – in two or three sessions – but then kept losing what she had gained by carrying heavy shopping and going back to work too early.

Ironically, but understandably, nurses suffer a high rate of low-back pain. A survey carried out in hospitals by chiropractors* showed that the highest incidence of back pain and injury was among the younger nurses (49 per cent suffering their first episode before the age of twenty-five), particularly in geriatric wards. Although nurses are shown correct ways of lifting during their training, conditions in busy wards don't necessarily allow them to take care of their own bodies while lifting other people's. Nurses with back strain are usually prescribed rest and physiotherapy, but chiropractors believe that this is often not enough; the

*'A study of back pain in nurses' by A. C. Breen, D.C., and S. G. Lloyd, D.C., *European Journal of Chiropractic*, March 1985.

spine may also need adjustment. Once a nurse's back has been weakened problems are liable to recur and worsen, forcing many to leave the profession early. Chiropractors feel that both the suffering and the wastage of trained staff could be prevented if chiropractic treatment could be given immediately after the first injury.

It says much for the efficacy of chiropractic that some women chiropractors, including Susan Moore and Alison Gordon-Creed, suffered severe back problems themselves before taking up a profession that involves continual standing, bending and lifting. They both recognize the importance of not working longer hours than is good for them, and getting regular preventative treatment. Susan's first job was in a very busy practice, and 'after five years, although I was only twenty-seven, my back was in a worse state than most of my patients'. So I decided to take my own advice.' Although she doesn't like doing exercises she built her strength up slowly with isometric exercises, and now weight-trains in a gym two or three times a week for overall fitness and especially to keep her back and stomach muscles toned up. She also limits her working hours to what she has found to be optimum for her back. She is now, she says, fitter than she has ever been.

CHAPTER SIX

TREATING CHILDREN

Children and even small babies can benefit from chiropractic, not only for musculo-skeletal problems, but for some Type O problems too, including colic, constipation and bed-wetting. Many problems stem from a difficult birth; a forceps delivery is very traumatic for the vulnerable neck and skull and even a normal birth puts a strain on the infant's neck. Although the bones are not properly formed at birth, stresses in the soft tissue can develop into spinal problems as the baby grows. In fact, in researching this chapter and the previous one I have been struck by just how many health problems, both emotional and physical, coincide with neck problems; in children they are often found alongside behavioural difficulties, asthma and allergies. Of course there is a chicken-and-egg situation here, since stress can also cause neck tension. But I can't help wondering how many difficulties might be avoided if it were standard practice for babies to have an expert spinal check-up, particularly after a difficult or prolonged birth.

Incautious handling at birth can also create other joint problems. The obstetrician who parts the infant's legs over-energetically to examine it may cause a rotated hip leading to a short leg and foot-dragging, and even occasionally to dislocation of the hip joint which may not be noticed at the time. It may be possible to treat the latter chiropractically, without resort to surgery; at least one chiropractor has successfully treated congenital hip dislocation in babies a few months old.

As children grow, they are susceptible to falls and bumps which can jar the growing spine. It is usual to think of children as bouncy, resilient creatures, for whom falls are a normal part of growing up. But growing bones and joints are vulnerable, and no chiropractor would regard a mother as being over-anxious if she brought her child in for a check-up after a heavy fall, even if no bones were broken. Bad posture, sitting at school desks, or lounging in front of the TV can also lead to early disc degeneration. Chiropractors are constantly seeing adult patients whose troubles have built up unnecessarily since childhood.

Some chiropractors have a special interest in treating children, but any well-trained practitioner knows how to apply gentle techniques that will not hurt or alarm a child; not every chiropractor would treat small babies, however, since their musculo-skeletal systems require specialist techniques. Below are some examples of ailments for which it would be worth consulting a chiropractor. A reputable practitioner will examine the child and tell you whether a spinal dysfunction is involved, which can be adjusted. If factors like diet play a part in the condition, the chiropractor will check whether these have been looked into, and may suggest changes where appropriate.

Infant Colic

This might not seem an obvious candidate for manipulation but, as we have seen, disorders of the gut may well relate to a vertebral problem. Madeleine Brzeski, a McTimoney chiropractor who treats a lot of children, successfully treated a case after the mother had tried all the dietary possibilities. When Madeleine examined the baby, she found a problem in the neck. 'When I adjusted it, it felt as if a ripple went through the baby's body as it relaxed; it was obviously holding a lot of tension there – it had had quite a difficult birth.'

In 1984 the Danish Chiropractors Association carried out a study by means of a questionnaire on infant chiropractic patients, with the aim of finding out for which ailments infants below the age of twelve months were taken to chiropractors. Of the 189 (out of 270) parents who responded, 132 had brought their babies (with an average age of six weeks) with infant colic. Of these, 72 (54 per cent) were cured, and 48 (37 per cent) improved; 12 (9 per cent) showed no change, and none was worse. The change in symptoms occurred after an average of two to three treatments, showing that this was not a case of the disease 'burning out'. Even if the 30 per cent of parents who didn't reply were not helped, this is still a high rate of cure. Dr Niels Nilsson, a medical doctor as well as a chiropractor, reported on this study in the *European Journal of Chiropractic* (December 1985). He writes: 'While this study does not prove that manipulation is the most efficient treatment for infant colic, it does certainly raise the question.' A more detailed and scientifically constructed study is currently being conducted.

Asthma, Bronchial Disorders and Allergy

Children with asthmatic and respiratory disorders often respond very well to chiropractic treatment. One chiropractor recalls developing asthma himself at the age of eleven; a single adjustment cleared it up completely. Several treatments are more usually needed for a complete cure. The New Zealand Commission was told of a two-year-old with severe asthma, who seemed to be getting worse under medical care. In desperation his parents took him to a chiropractor who did not promise a cure, but examined the child and suggested, correctly, that he might have had a fall at some time. After the child's neck had been adjusted there was a dramatic improvement; his constant wheeze almost vanished and he had his first uninterrupted night's sleep for a long time. After further treatments over a few months, the asthma had completely gone. This kind of case will be familiar to many chiropractors. It certainly makes theoretical sense to free the child's nervous system to function fully, rather than loading the body with drugs which can make it drowsy, slow down the metabolic rate, and possibly affect its eating habits as well.

Hyperactivity, Behavioural and Nervous Disorders

If a happy child below the age of speech suddenly becomes fractious and difficult, this may be his only way of telling you that he has a pain or headache. A spinal examination may be well worth while, particularly if the child has had a fall before the change in behaviour. Falls can also lead to altered behaviour and uncharacteristic aggressiveness in older children, especially if the neck has been affected.

Hyperactivity, unfortunately increasingly common these days, is generally associated with a reaction to foods and food additives. When examined by chiropractors, hyperactive children are often found to have an abnormally large number of spinal problems as well. Whether these cause the hyperactivity or are caused by it is not known, but treating them often helps to calm children down. As with asthma, the biomechanical factor may be one element in the whole syndrome, and when that element is dealt with the child stands a much better chance of coping.

Susan Moore sees quite a few hyperactive children. 'I don't claim to be able to cure them, but I check the whole spine out and if I find anything wrong I'll treat it and see if it makes any difference. In most cases it does. Hyperactive children have a lot of neck and low-back problems, which can affect their behaviour, especially the neck – a lot of hyperactive children have had a stressful birth. Of course many of them have been found to have various food allergies, but diet doesn't necessarily control the whole thing. A lot of those I see bed-wet as well, which seems to come from the low back. So whatever's wrong, I treat the whole spine in the same session.'

Many of these young patients respond very well. In one case a desperate mother brought in her eight-year-old daughter who was suffering from lack of co-ordination, reading difficulties, hyperactivity and bed-wetting; in seven treatments she improved considerably. Interestingly, the mother wasn't convinced that her improvement related to the spine. Then, after a fall, the child's behaviour reverted to what it had been before, and once again it settled after chiropractic treatment. This time the mother acknowledged that the treatment was responsible.

One unhappy thirteen-year-old was brought to Madeleine Brzeski with the dire label 'non-specific neurological deficiency syndrome'. She had a reading age of four, was overweight, aggressive and violent, and lacked sufficient co-ordination even to dress herself. After a few treatments Madeleine put her on a sugar- and additive-free diet, which brought about an immediate weight loss, and made her look and feel much more attractive. Madeleine did a lot of cranial work on her, manipulating the bones of the face and skull, as well as working on her very curved spine. Her behavioural problems settled down; she became relaxed and started sleeping well. After about nine months of treatment her reading age was ten; she could dance, skip – and use a computer. And she can look forward to being an integrated member of society.

Bed-wetting and Bladder Problems

As mentioned above, bed-wetting may relate to the lumbar area of the spine, affecting the nerve supply to the bladder. Children suffering from low-back pain following a fall often bed-wet as a side-effect, and both can be treated simultaneously. Madeleine Brzeski has treated several such children. She told me: 'Only one child has come specifically for bed-wetting, a six-year-old who was becoming very embarrassed about it, because she wanted to stay with friends. She had a pelvic problem, and after two treatments she was fine.'

Other urinary problems may also respond to chiropractic. Susan Moore treated an eleven-year-old girl who had been feeling generally unwell for two months, with a frequent need to pass water. No medical cause had been found. Examination showed that she was developing a slight scoliosis, and had mechanical joint fixations in the low back, mid thoracic and especially in the cervical vertebra; the last probably related to a strenuous forceps delivery. Susan treated all the areas affected and within two treatments the girl had improved dramatically. Although this was followed by ups and downs, especially with the bladder problems, everything had cleared up within a year.

Vision and Hearing

Defects in vision and hearing can stem from so many causes that it would be irresponsible to suggest a chiropractic check-up in all cases. However, when there is definitely a vertebral problem cures and improvements, though rare, do occur. The connection may not always be obvious. John McTimoney treated a twelve-year-old who had become deaf following mumps at the age of two; after six weekly treatments she was able to throw away the hearing aid she had had to wear for three years.

A New Zealand woman had a daughter who suffered from impaired hearing, and an ear, nose and throat specialist recommended surgery. The mother decided to try chiropractic first; the day following an adjustment to the neck the child's hearing became normal. The specialist, though amazed at the improvement, remarked: 'Of course if you are going to do this sort of thing you might get temporary relief but you will have her back here within six months.' Fortunately he was wrong; the girl, now grown-up, has perfect hearing.

Even more striking is the case of a girl of nine who was diagnosed as having retinitis pigmentosa – chronic progressive degeneration of the retina, narrowing the field of vision. Her mother, who was already a patient of Brian Carter, a BCA chiropractor, was naturally extremely depressed at the prospect of her child losing her sight. One day the little girl's vision seemed to improve following a fall in the playground; the mother mentioned this to Brian Carter and he offered to examine her spine to see if there was any correlation. He found a very marked fixation in the joints of the neck, which needed adjustment, although it was impossible to say that this was the cause of the eye problem. After the first treatment there was a marked increase in the child's visual range, and after a total of four treatments at monthly intervals her eyesight was normal again. This is the kind of case that the medical profession often dismisses as impossible and therefore it must have been 'misdiagnosed' – indeed, on the little girl's next visit to the eye hospital the child was at first accused of lying. However, tests showed that her visual range was now wider than her mother's; moreover, she had been seen by two different specialists, each of whom had already confirmed the other's diagnosis.

Still's Disease

This is a painful and disabling form of inflammatory arthritis in children; chiropractic treatment should only be sought with the cooperation of the doctor in charge of the case. Madeleine Brzeski recounted what struck me as a remarkable instance of medical open-mindedness. (The consultant concerned, motivated by what was best for his patient, doesn't consider it particularly remarkable.) When thirteen-year-old Stephen Coleman fell ill with the disease his mother, hearing that Madeleine had had some success with rheumatoid arthritis, spoke to the consultant paediatrician, Dr H. Marcovitch, and he invited Madeleine in for a talk about her work.

The management of Still's Disease includes the use of anti-inflammatory drugs during the acute phase; ensuring that the child's joints become as little deformed as possible (which involves protecting the limbs with splints and plaster casts): and finally, once the acute pain and discomfort has died down, restoring mobility to the joints and strength to the wasted muscles. It was in this last area that Dr Marcovitch felt that Madeleine could help, particularly as she was offering her services unpaid, and the amount of time she was prepared to give seemed preferable to his other options, which were three short sessions of physiotherapy a week, or the boy's removal to a distant hospital. Having discussed her work with her he decided that she would be an excellent person to help with this problem.

Madeleine started working with Stephen while he was going through the inflammatory stage of the disease. He was given conventional medication and was in plaster for a short time, but the hospital allowed Madeleine to help reduce the inflammation with cold compresses rather than by using their hot wax treatment. They also cooperated with her suggestion of putting him on a special diet, free of sugar, additives and red meat, and introduced her to the physiotherapist who taught her the remedial exercises she would normally have carried out. Instead of having to be sent to a special hospital the boy was sent home under Madeleine's care. She treated him for just over a year, using the very gentle McTimoney techniques every day at first.

By the end of the year his blood tests were clear, he had very little joint deformity, and was able to return to school. He started playing rugby again, against Madeleine's better judgement, and the disease returned. Madeleine treated him again, in conjunction with the local GP and the hospital; all three kept in communication, and the boy recovered once more.

It is impossible to say for certain whether the child did better with chiropractic care than he would otherwise have done. Certainly, comments the GP cautiously, Madeleine supplied moral support for the family, who felt something was being done for their child. Dr Marcovitch says that the boy, who had relatively severe acute Still's Disease when he presented, recovered remarkably well. 'One can't say whether chiropractic was better than conventional physiotherapy or not, because it's not been tested out in any numbers,' he says, 'but simple common sense would suggest that the amount of time she was able to offer would be better than anything I could organize under the NHS.' Madeleine tells me she would like the opportunity to treat more such cases with medical cooperation.

Scoliosis

Slight scoliosis, an S-shaped curve in the spine seen from the back, can easily occur in growing children as a result of poor posture, and even of the strain of activities like ballet classes. The sooner it is treated the better; although some people have scoliosis with no pain or difficulties, it may develop into much more serious problems as the child grows. Very severe cases may unfortunately need hospital treatment (such as plaster corsets or even surgery). A chiropractor will be able to tell whether this is necessary or whether he can treat the case himself.

Accidents, Injuries, Aches and Pains

Chiropractors often find themselves dealing with the results of school sports and games, such as ankle injuries and peripheral joint strains. Most would like the opportunity to do more preventative work. This may consist of simply checking technical faults in their training, or seeing that there are no congenital problems which could make the child unsuitable for heavy athletic training. Some parents can be over-ambitious for their children's sporting prowess, and while the musculo-skeletal system is still developing there is a risk of causing long-term damage in straining the growing joints and ligaments by over-exertion. In fact any aches, pains or back-aches in a child, whether athletic or not, should never be dismissed as 'growing pains'; there is always a reason for pain.

More than one chiropractor has adopted the profession as a result of childhood injury. At the age of thirteen, on holiday abroad, Ian Hutchinson had a severe fall down a thirty-foot river bank and was hospitalized for a week with severe bruises and grazes, although no bones were broken. But on returning to school he suffered from neck and back pain, and brief blackouts. Doctors were unable to help, but eventually a chiropractor cured him completely. Later, he was considering a career in medicine when he met the chiropractor again and got talking. 'It struck me that there were so many people medicine hadn't been able to help, yet nearly all of them had been helped by chiropractic; I felt that chiropractic was something more valuable to go in for.'

Susan Moore also switched from an intended medical career after chiropractic had helped her with a long-term and increasingly disabling back problem. She speaks from experience: 'When children develop back problems and they are not treated straight away, especially during the teenage years when they're growing, the weaknesses grow with them and they are left with problems that will flare up for the rest of their lives.' Her own problems began with low-back pain at the age of thirteen; physiotherapy, heat and massage gave temporary relief, but the pain always returned and, as the years went by, travelled up her spine, causing headaches and neck pains as well. Sitting was extremely painful – and at school one has to sit all day; taking O- and A-levels was a miserable experience. Over five years Susan saw a number of different specialists, whose final conclusion was: 'You've got back trouble; we don't know why. You'll have to be on pain-killers for the rest of your life.'

'At seventeen, going on eighteen, that seemed ridiculous,' says Susan. 'When some friends suggested chiropractic, my mother took me in sheer desperation. Chiropractic didn't get me totally right, but it gave me my first constant relief – and the chiropractor found out the cause. I was a very keen swimmer and swam butterfly up to County standard. *Now* I know that I have a hypermobile spine; the joints are much more flexible than they should be, which means you can strain the ligaments and muscles around them much more easily than the normal person. This can lead to joint problems and the joints lock; if you're not fit, that can happen with increasing regularity. Doing butterfly I was arching the back all the time, which my spine wasn't basically built to do. The funny thing was that all those specialists used to say, "You swim? Great, carry on!" But they never asked what stroke I did. By the time I got to see the chiropractor I'd given up swimming because my back was so bad.

'I was so impressed with what chiropractic had done for me that although I'd already got a place in medical school I decided to switch to chiropractic instead. I was already doing A-level science, which I needed to go to the Anglo-European College. I wouldn't say I was disillusioned by medicine, but my experience as a patient was that orthodox medicine didn't have all the answers.'

Alison Gordon-Creed is convinced that preventative chiropractic treatment when young would have saved her a spinal operation and its consequences; she has an interest in treating babies and children preventatively, and some mothers are bringing her their children for check-ups rather than waiting till they develop serious problems. Some McTimoney patients who have been treated preventatively since childhood believe they have better over-all health than their contemporaries.

Preventative treatment shouldn't be carried too far, of course. I'm told by British chiropractors that they are sometimes asked to treat American visitors whose spines have been manipulated so often that their joints are completely loose and there is really nothing to adjust. As Susan Moore's story shows, loose joints don't necessarily mean a healthy spine. The British way is to adjust simply when and where it is needed, and not to suggest weekly return visits for years. But I have yet to meet a chiropractor who wouldn't rather give preventative treatment to a child in slight pain than have a queue of unnecessarily disabled patients at his door.

CHAPTER SEVEN

CHIROPRACTIC

FOR ANIMALS

The Legal Position

In Britain, legislation on the treatment of animals is much more stringent than that which applies to human beings. Under the Veterinary Surgeons Act, only qualified veterinary surgeons are allowed to diagnose and treat animals, on the principle that while humans can look after themselves, animals need protection – though dog-owners and farmers are allowed to treat their own animals, provided they don't practise surgery. It is possible, however, for physiotherapy and manipulation to be practised on animals under the supervision of a vet, and a few chiropractors work with vets on this basis. Animals, like humans, can develop spinal and other problems for which chiropractic is appropriate, and some vets are happy to refer their clients to practitioners whom they know to be suitably skilled and qualified.

Like the medical profession, the veterinary profession has become more open-minded over recent years and alternative therapies like homoeopathy, acupuncture and manipulation have gained some acceptance among them. Some vets practise various forms of manipulation themselves, while others who recognize its possibilities use it as another tool to offer to clients, particularly those who are reluctant to over-medicate their animals.

As the law now stands, using a chiropractor involves owners in a double fee, since they have to pay the vet for a diagnosis first. There must be a strong temptation on the part of the animal-owners to make direct contact with local chiropractors whose work they know, by-passing the veterinary diagnosis – and a strong temptation for the chiropractor to agree. Stuart Hastie, a vet who worked with John McTimoney in the 1960s, is anxious to promote good relations between the veterinary and paramedical professions; he himself manipulates horses, using some of McTimoney's techniques. But he is concerned that some chiropractors may be treating animals without veterinary supervision. 'There are very few cases where a horse's back "goes out" in McTimoney's sense, and very few of those where there is not some other primary condition, whether it be the rider, the fit of the saddle, bad teeth, navicular disease of the front feet, or bad riding techniques. Chiropractors, qualified or unqualified, may fail to pick up these related conditions which are so relevant. I work on the basis that only a third of cases treated with chiropractic do any good to any extent.'

How far Mr Hastie's fears are justified is hard to judge. Mr Tim Moore, a vet and horse-owner, is very happy to use McTimoney chiropractors. 'I have top-level international eventers of my own, and I know from results that, having had a back corrected, the horse then comes right. That doesn't mean to say that if there's been an abnormality for some time the back won't slip out again.'

McTimoney-trained chiropractors would claim a success rate of nearer 80 per cent than Mr Hastie's 33 per cent; and their training should enable them to preclude conditions which are not treatable chiropractically. (They also say that since animals appear to have fewer psychological problems than human beings, they heal more quickly!) Unfortunately no trials have been carried out to measure the success rate or diagnostic abilities of McTimoney or BCA chiropractors in relation to animals. Meanwhile, the law stands; for chiropractors to treat animals lawfully without the participation of vets a statutory instrument would need to be passed by government. John McTimoney hoped to achieve this in his lifetime but ill-health forced him to abandon the project (see page 171).

Dogs with Disc Problems

Where a good relationship exists between chiropractor and vet, treatment in appropriate cases can be extremely beneficial. All kinds of dogs, for instance, can get disc problems; particularly prone are long-backed dogs like dachshunds and basset hounds – nicknamed by vets 'suspension bridges on legs'. 'Slipped discs' can paralyse their hind legs: you sometimes see them getting about on little trolleys. Vets generally take X-rays to determine where the problem is, and if possible prescribe 'conservative treatment' similar to that applied to human beings, consisting of rest and painkillers. Most dogs with disc problems recover naturally, though those in intractable pain may need prompt surgery. But there is another option. Chiropractic can bring about recoveries that are both remarkably swift and permanent, even when there are calcified vertebrae. A number of chiropractors have successfully treated dogs, including paraplegic dachshunds, and once a vet has experienced the benefits of chiropractic on his canine patients he will refer suitable cases.

George Walker, for instance, has a good relationship with local vet Nigel Taylor, who told me: 'A few years ago we had two dogs with disc problems who were not responding well to conventional treatment – a rough collie and a Cavalier King Charles spaniel. Neither of the owners were keen on surgery or further medication, and one of the other vets in my practice suggested getting in touch with George. What impressed me as a clinician was that he was able to pinpoint accurately where the problem was before being shown the X-ray, and I decided to give it a try. He manipulated the spaniel on two or three occasions and she made a satisfactory recovery with no need for medication. The collie had cervical disc problems, and was really paraplegic. George manipulated it at our request and within forty-eight hours it was walking. After that, the practice started using him whenever appropriate.

'Every vet is different – we know George, and a lot of our clients go to him for themselves, so we can offer them this unique service. My problem is to be sure that chiropractic is the best answer, or whether an animal needs surgery or medication. For the dog with a bad back or non-specific lameness which I am unable to control with medication, it can offer a half-way house between surgery, which is fairly traumatic for the animal, and giving up on the case.'

John McTimoney's Magic Fingers

John McTimoney was by no means the first person to manipulate animals, but he claimed that his system was 'the first application of chiropractic in a complete form for animals'. It started in 1953 when one of McTimoney's patients cancelled an appointment as the vet was coming to shoot his seven-year-old mare, which for some months had had a swollen fetlock that would not respond to treatment. McTimoney, thinking this might be the effect of a sub-luxated vertebra, offered to look at her. As he wrote: 'Trained in human anatomy and with farming experience I adapted my knowledge of the human anatomy to that of the animal and worked out a method of adjusting the vertebrae which were subluxated ... and cured the horse in two weeks. By the end of the month the horse ... was hunting again and continued to do so for many years. At the age of twenty-one she was in foal.'

McTimoney further refined and adapted his techniques, and by 1964 was known for curing all types of disorders after normal veterinary methods had failed to help – lameness, lack of co-ordination, and bucking and shying in horses, and lameness and 'slipped discs' in dogs. For ten years he ran into no real conflict with the veterinary profession; most vets were not interested in his work.

Then in 1964, after an article had appeared in a local paper about his cure of a bulldog with eczema, the Royal College of Veterinary Surgeons wrote to McTimoney pointing out that he was breaking the law by practising veterinary surgery, and could be prosecuted. McTimoney replied that he was not practising veterinary surgery but an entirely new system of animal chiropractic by which he had treated animals for ten years with remarkable results. He invited them to investigate his work, but the invitation was not taken up. Meanwhile his solicitors obtained a letter from the RCVS saying that they were prepared to regard chiropractors as physiotherapists, who are granted an exemption from the law provided they work under and with a vet.

As a result of the publicity, however, one vet did show an interest – Mr E. Herrod-Taylor, M.R.C.V.S., now a well-known name in the field of animal manipulation. He was the first to appreciate the potential of animal chiropractic and became good friends with McTimoney. He worked with him on a number of horses and became a proficient chiropractor himself. He too tried to interest the veterinary profession, but met with little success. Nevertheless he helped to train further McTimoney chiropractors, and until recently taught at the MCS; sadly, this work was cut short by a stroke, and I have been unable to interview him.

McTimoney's other veterinary ally, Stuart Hastie, 'became interested in what he was doing with some of my cases – with or without my consultation. If I don't understand something I want to know what's going on, and he and I became quite good friends eventually. But he persisted in treating animals without a veterinary diagnosis, which set a pattern that worries me from the aspect of our relationship with the paramedical world.'

McTimoney continued his efforts to interest the veterinary establishment in the potential of chiropractic, not as a method of veterinary surgery but as 'a new method which can help in cases where there is not a response to normal methods, apart from the fact that normal methods of veterinary surgery cannot help to improve the gait, movement, co-ordination, style or vices of the horse, which is what has been achieved with my methods'. But in the 1960s the general opinion was that it was impossible to manipulate a horse's spine, and that the whole thing smacked of charlatanism. In 1967 he visited the RCVS to show them a film of his work; this seems to have met with a stunning lack of response.* (It is depressing, in the history of chiropractic and other alternative therapies, how often the response to the unknown is 'This is impossible, therefore we will not even look at it', rather than 'This person appears to be doing something interesting, let's have a look!')

Impossible or not, McTimoney's techniques became very popular with horse-owners and show-jumpers, and today the British royal household has its horses treated by McTimoney-trained chiropractors, one of whom is flown to various exotic places to treat the animals of other wealthy horse-owners.

McTimoney's own clients included professional riders like Dorian Williams and David Broome. 'I was one of Mr McTimoney's greatest fans,' David Broome recalls. 'He was a masterpiece. A lot of people follow him and do it as well, but that guy was something special. He did my own back, and you felt something was happening when he touched you, something about the touch of his fingers was different from anybody else's.

'He worked wonders on Beethoven, the horse I won the World Championships on; he was going very badly one day and I took him to McTimoney. He gave him one treatment,

*This interesting film, entitled 'Spinal Manipulation for Horses' (18 minutes, colour; heading: Veterinary), is in the library of the National Film Archives.

he just knew what was going wrong. He said, "Don't jump him for four days", and I jumped him on the fifth day at the Dublin Show, and he won the first two classes he entered. The man was a gem, and a gentleman with it.'

With fans like this, it is not surprising that the demand for animal treatment, as well as for his human practice, became so great that McTimoney's heart eventually gave out. He suffered his first heart attack in 1969. He had just started an action to change the law and Quintin Hogg, now Lord Hailsham, had agreed to represent him; but because of his illness and the expense involved in legal action he decided regretfully to withdraw, though still convinced that 'no veterinary surgeon is qualified or conversant enough with my method to be able to give me direction or prescription and would not know when I should be called in'.

When he started his school in 1972 he included animal chiropractic in the course. Students were faced with all kinds of animals, including sheep, and their studies were not without moments of humour. One current joke was: 'How do you adjust a Jack Russell?', the answer being, 'Bloody quickly!' Unfortunately the students never carried out their plan to hire a boa constrictor from a zoo and seat it in McTimoney's waiting-room.

Some dozen McTimoney chiropractors are now qualified to treat animals under veterinary supervision, and more are on the way. After a break, the course was resumed in 1986 as an extension to the main course, open to MCS graduates only; the curriculum includes a lecture on the law given by the solicitor who dealt with McTimoney's correspondence with the RCVS.

How Do You Manipulate a Horse?

Whether you *should* manipulate a horse depends, as with human beings, on the diagnosis. Whether you *can* do so no longer seems to be in question; thinking has changed since the 1960s, and a number of people in the horse world practise physiotherapy and other manipulative techniques, as well as chiropractic. McTimoney's complete system involves adjusting most of the joints, including the pelvis, and a specific adjustment to the atlas, the first cervical bone just behind the head. (Interestingly, in view of the effects of adjusting the neck in human beings, this technique can also calm a nervous animal.) Some vets still question adjustment of the spine itself: they believe a horse's spine is extremely solid.

A report by L. B. Jeffcott and G. Dalin published in the *Equine Veterinary Journal* in 1980 concludes, from experimental studies on five fresh *post mortem* thoroughbreds, that the maximum possible movement of an individual spinous process is 1.1–6 mm, and that from an anatomical viewpoint 'the so-called vertebral subluxation ... appears to be a misnomer and may simply be attributable to muscular imbalance leading to a spastic scoliosis'. The authors comment that although the results of chiropractic manipulation of horses with back problems are reported to be dramatic and instantaneous, the incidence of recurrence of symptoms is, apparently, high. It is possible, they say, that the effect of sharp pressure on the spinous processes relaxes the muscles that are held in tension, improving the horse's performance. 'However, this is only a tentative theory and the whole matter needs further investigation before it can be satisfactorily resolved.'

There are several horror-stories circulating about people (always unnamed) using mallets* to 'knock back' a horse's

*Seventy-year-old Ronnie Longford of Pebworth trained with McTimoney after being helped with his own back injuries, and has become one of the best-known animal manipulators in the UK and abroad. Since his hands have been affected by arthritis he has developed a technique for manipulation using a miniature mallet (about 1½ inches in diameter) for adjustments that he is unable to carry out manually. Perhaps this is the origin of the 'mallet' rumour; if so, it demonstrates again how much better it would be if people would investigate what is actually happening instead of drawing the worst conclusions!

vertebra, or swinging from beams to move them with their feet! A report in *Horse and Pony* (November 1978) describes how a piece of bone was actually kicked off the vertebra of an unfortunate horse treated in this fashion by a 'quack'; the same report claims that spinal manipulation is impossible in horses, and that equine disc problems are incurable. Based on that example alone, such a conclusion is understandable, if limited. Conversely, some people might wonder how the McTimoney techniques, which can be remarkably light and gentle, can have any effect at all.

Mr Bob Bainbridge, who kindly drew my attention to the report quoted above, is information officer of the Equine Veterinary Association. He told me: 'We keep an open mind on it. Jeffcott's study concluded that it was physically impossible to move one vertebra upon another in the main part of the spinal column; it would require greater strength than a man could exert. But that may be the principle on which chiropractic, as opposed to manipulation, does work, because chiropractors don't use strength to re-position vertebrae, they set about using blocks of muscle one against another, and stimulating muscle. What must be questioned from a scientific point of view is how they actually achieve their results, and this is very difficult to evaluate. I'm open-minded, but no one has adequately explained what they do.' In fact IPC chiropractors claim that the recoil action created by a McTimoney-style adjustment is based on good engineering principles of leverage.

Lynda Clark, a McTimoney chiropractor in her thirties, manipulates horses among other animals referred to her by vets – all nine stone and five foot five of her. The secret, she explained to me, lies in the speed and angle of the adjustment, and not in brute force. 'Obviously if I were to try and pit my strength against even a Shetland pony I wouldn't win. It works because you are using their strength to help you instead of trying to beat it. If you do an adjustment on the back really fast you see a muscle reaction a split second afterwards, which helps the adjustment. Usually you get a bounce reaction in the back; someone once watching the whole thing from a distance told me the head did a nod as well – the whole body moved!'

McTimoney chiropractors say that on palpation the spinous processes can feel as much as half an inch out of alignment, but, as in humans, the misalignment is frequently very subtle. Misalignments as small as a millimetre are still very important, since they can affect the transmission of nerve impulses. Also as with humans, McTimoney chiropractors take a 'whole body' approach, working on all the animal's joints as well as on the spine.

Horses apparently have their own ways of telling you they have back-ache. 'It's usually a change of temperament, like starting to refuse jumps,' says Lynda, 'or a very placid horse who suddenly won't have his head touched, or is miserable and bad-tempered. Some animals doing athletic things will put in stops where they never would before, as if they were saying, "No, that's going to hurt me – I'm not going to do it." Or they start to go a bit to one side of a jump instead of in the middle. With dressage anything wrong with the back shows up quite quickly, because they move in a different way to accommodate it. Most horses are very good about being adjusted. Some are a bit skittish when you first start and calm down during treatment.'

Although there seems to be some doubt as regards the manipulation of horses, it is clearly appropriate under the right conditions and with the right sort of expectations. Veterinary surgeon Tim Moore, who uses chiropractors regularly, says: 'My interpretation of what a chiropractor does is this: there is a misalignment in the spine, usually fractional; they don't necessarily put the bone back, but they set up a vibration which causes the bone to correct itself, if the muscles will allow it to correct. I believe in chiropractic, as a horse-owner as well as a veterinary surgeon. There are still a number of veterinary surgeons that

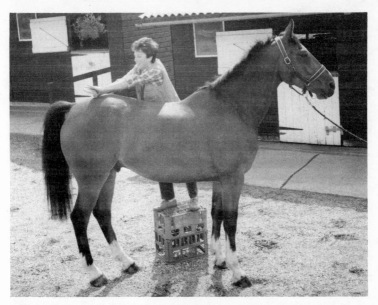

**'Most horses are very good about being adjusted.' An animal
chiropractor at work**

don't believe in it; all I can say is they should try using
chiropractors and see. I wouldn't ask my clients to try anything that I hadn't tried myself.'

An Animal Chiropractor's Work

How does someone set about developing a legitimate career
as an animal chiropractor? Lynda Clark told me her story.
'I had always wanted to work with animals, but was guided
into secretarial work by my parents. Seven years ago I saw
an advert for the school in Banbury, and went along, not
knowing anything about chiropractic at all. I had had
osteopathic treatment myself and was fascinated to discover
how manipulation could be applied to animals, so I joined
the course; we had to learn on people first. It certainly

works, it's marvellous. Obviously it's not a panacea for all ills, but where it is indicated it can be fantastic.

'When I started practice I was very unsure of myself and worried because I'd heard that vets could be very anti-chiropractic. I started with people, and did a little animal work if I was asked, but didn't go out looking for it. Every time an animal came up I made sure the owner let their vet know and got his permission, and I would report back to the vet. Now I work with one vet in particular, and a number of others too, occasionally. As my confidence has grown, so has the practice.

'I mainly treat horses, but I get a fair number of dogs – including recently a police dog; they work quite hard, and have to jump huge heights in their training. His gait was most peculiar, and his handler was worried he would have to retire him early, but he seems to be going on all right since I treated him. No significant abnormality showed up on his X-rays, although there was said to be some "wear and tear". In my terms the pelvis was not correctly aligned and this chiropractically could account for the wear and tear and his peculiar gait.

'I treat farm animals – sheep, cows, goats, rams. A male colleague has treated a couple of bulls; they get back trouble covering cows! Rams can have similar trouble; both rams and bulls can slip, and bulls who fall on to concrete yards get back problems and don't want to get on with it!'

The sex life of animals seems fraught with unusual perils. Lynda was also brought a drake: 'He had had an X-ray, and the vet said he had dislocated his neck and he couldn't really do anything with it. He seems to have got his head stuck in some netting going after his female companion, and twisted to pull it out, and he came in looking at the world upside down. I treated him and in a few days he gradually started to get right. So I don't know if I can claim to have done it or if time did it!

'I've also treated a couple of cats. One, the owner told

me, was getting old and arthritic, she'd had a few litters, and could no longer jump in and out of the window. When I felt her, her pelvis was rotated slightly, and I adjusted that. Next morning the owner phoned and said, "She's just jumped in through the window." Which was lovely! Quite often people say afterwards, "I didn't like to tell you, but I thought you were going to have trouble." But she didn't mind being adjusted; they very rarely do, funnily enough.'

PART FOUR

THE FUTURE OF CHIROPRACTIC

Extract from a conversation with two AECC students:
FIRST STUDENT: 'It's so much fun – the thrill of seeing people improve! Very often we're their last hope.'
SECOND STUDENT: 'I don't like the thought of being the last hope of the destitute!'

In 1976 Dr David Owen, then Minister of State for Health, set up a Working Group on back pain under the chairmanship of Professor A. L. Cochrane. Its report, published in 1979, concluded that back pain was widespread, unpleasant and at times serious, that existing services for its relief were variable in quality and availability and indeterminate in effectiveness, that there was a profound and widespread dissatisfaction with available treatment on offer, but that evidence on available treatment was unsatisfactory and often conflicting. It urged the need for more research in order to provide more effective treatment.

In 1986 back pain is still a national problem, and the services offered by conventional medicine have not been improved by cuts in NHS funding. GPs themselves recognize that they are not doing a great job as far as backs are concerned. Yet people who have undergone a serious training in spinal problems and are skilled in their treatment have to work outside the medical profession as 'alternative practitioners'.

Chiropractic in Britain has not suffered as it has in other countries from the antagonism of the medical profession; a good many doctors and a few orthopaedic surgeons already refer patients to both chiropractors and osteopaths, and use them themselves. Even the report, *Alternative Therapy*, published by the British Medical Association in May 1986, a generally skimpy and shallow overview of alternative therapies, allowed that in the field of manipulation properly trained and registered lay practitioners could provide a safe and helpful service. But at present that service is limited by financial considerations and availability.

Paying for Health

The existence of the NHS has accustomed the British public to 'free' medical treatment (we tend to forget that we are actually paying for it). To visit a chiropractor regularly for some months can be a financial burden, even though most chiropractors' fees seem reasonable enough, particularly in comparison with private medicine. One or two doctors and surgeons have suggested that chiropractors and osteopaths are making fortunes from their patients' gullibility; I doubt whether many fortunes are made, and I doubt whether many people would choose to go through a four-year training (often financed by themselves) in order to spend their working lives treating people's bodies, without a genuine concern for people and an interest in healing bodies. The fact that they *want* to enter the NHS is an indication of their concern for people's welfare.

As a matter of interest, George Walker tells me that the conflict which the British experience in paying for health care takes place on both sides of the therapist's desk; having had chiropractors of many nationalities working at his clinic, he has observed that the British have a peculiar problem in charging *enough* for their services. He adds that often those patients who ask for concessions are those who don't really need them, while those who do may be sacrificing a great deal to pay for treatment.

The obvious, if far from simple, answer would be to make the services of chiropractors and other properly qualified manipulators available on the NHS, and this is one of the declared aims of the BCA. For acceptance by the medical authorities, research is needed to show that patients actually benefit, and some is already under way. Meanwhile the public is voting with its feet, and its purse. Chiropractors are kept very busy. And since most people are not stupid enough to continue paying for what is of no benefit to them, one must conclude that chiropractors are helping them.

As we have seen, many patients come as a last resort, often after years of pain, some after surgical damage. In a country which is supposed to provide a 'Health Service' this seems ludicrous. James Rousseau is fond of quoting an advertisement he saw in the USA: 'Chiropractic first, drugs second, surgery last'; this sums up the views of most chiropractors. In many cases of back pain early intervention by an expert could save years of suffering – it would also surely reduce NHS costs in the long run. But as long as this kind of treatment is only available privately, even those doctors who are in favour of alternative therapies hesitate to refer patients until it is clear that conventional medicine cannot help them.

Dr Marcovitch, who was able to put a child patient into the care of a chiropractor only because she didn't charge (see page 160), voices what may be a widely held view. 'It is a great pity that the Health Service doesn't make more use of all these people. It's perfectly respectable for me to use a dietician or a physiotherapist, but there are other professions that I can't use, and I don't understand the logic ... I think that medicine hasn't faced up to a particular issue: medicine has to work out what are the things it can actually deal with very well, which we must keep our hands on because if anyone else took them over it might be a disaster, and what are the things for which it really doesn't have much to offer, like the treatment of low-back pain.'

Your Doctor and Your Back

Most chiropractors have built up good relationships with at least some GPs and surgeons. What about the rest?

Throughout the research for this book it has been sad to hear over and over again comments from patients like: 'My doctor wasn't interested', 'Doctors make me angry – ignoring people in genuine pain', 'I went to a chiropractor because I'd lost faith in conventional medicine.' Anna, whose sciatica was successfully treated by chiropractic, does not want her real name used because she works in a hospital. Her experience is probably typical. 'I couldn't discuss it with the doctor, he wasn't prepared to discuss it. He gave me a prescription and that was the end of the matter. I was very worried because it had been going on for months. I wanted some attention for it! It was very, very painful. He gave me a good examination and was satisfied in himself that whatever was wrong wasn't too severe. Maybe to him it was a discomfort, but to me it was a bad pain.' And a surgeon whose patients are often severely disabled and depressed by the time they reach him says: 'By the time they see me, they've seen ten people who've abandoned them anyway. The incidence of conventional medicine abandoning patients is most disturbing.'

There is still some lingering prejudice against manipulation, despite the fact that manipulation has been found to be much safer, in terms of reported damage, than either drugs or surgery. Some doctors are brusque with patients who ask for referral to a chiropractor or osteopath – or even a doctor who manipulates. Dr John Paterson, Vice-President and Hon. Secretary of the British Association of Manipulative Medicine, recalls that a few years ago one of his patients was told by her GP, 'Yes, go to him if you want to end up in a wheelchair!' The fear of such reactions means that numbers of patients don't tell their doctors when they visit alternative therapists. If doctors are really concerned about their patients' welfare more communication is needed between the two, rather than a cutting-off.

On the whole, the problem in Britain seems to be less one of prejudice than a simple lack of awareness of the availability and possibilities of spinal manipulation, of helplessness rather than heartlessness. Dr Drury, another doctor who would like to see alternative practitioners available on the NHS, points out: 'There is no doubt there is a group of patients, particularly with back pain, who get as frustrated with their doctors as their doctors get frustrated with them. Because it's pretty disillusioning seeing somebody for the twentieth time with the same pain and saying, "I'm sorry there is nothing more I can do for you."'

When a mature chiropractic student told his doctor that he was about to take the AECC training, the doctor replied, 'Good! Anything to get back pain out of my surgery!' And in the feasibility study for the trial to be run jointly by the MRC and the BCA at Northwick Park Hospital (of which more below) a hundred or so Harrow GPs were asked to state if they did not wish their patients to be entered: none took up the option, and several replied that the kind of study proposed was overdue, and offered their full cooperation.

Physiotherapists wish that doctors would refer more patients to experts in manipulation, of whatever school, instead of sending them home with pills and instructions to rest. 'It would help if members of the public told their GP, "Look, I'm not going to go away, please refer me to a chiropractor or whatever",' says Victoria Cichy of the Chartered Society of Physiotherapists. 'We are trying very hard to educate GPs in exactly what we do so that they know how and when to refer their patients. The problem is that once they find out we get flooded with patients!'

Some alternative practitioners fear that if their therapies are found to be medically acceptable the techniques will be adopted by doctors after an abbreviated training, ignoring

the philosophy underlying them and leaving the non-
medically trained therapists still outside the system. This
has already happened with acupuncture, which GPs can
practise after taking one weekend course. ('How would they
like it if I started prescribing drugs after one weekend
course?' asks a chiropractor.) In the case of manipulation,
this fear may not be justified; most doctors don't seem to be
very interested in practising it.

Medicine has developed separately from manipulation,
and in most medical schools there is an enormous gap in
training. Few doctors are taught to examine and palpate the
spine; the focus on academic rather than humane qualifications for entry into medical schools seems to have produced
a generation of doctors who don't particularly want to talk
to patients, let alone touch them. (Small wonder if people
turn to alternatives.) Efforts to introduce manipulative
techniques into medical training were made by the late Dr
James Cyriax of St Thomas's Hospital (where manipulation was and is taught), but although his lectures were
always crowded out, few doctors have followed them up.
(This may be as well, since from many accounts his teaching was limited, and not scientifically acceptable, and the
adjustments he taught have been described as painful and
clumsy.) Dr Cyriax was another pioneer figure in the field
of manipulation whose arrogance and outspokenness
antagonized many of his contemporaries, but in preaching
the need for experts in spinal care he was only talking sense.

In 1963 the British Association of Manipulative Medicine (BAMM) was founded, to bring together those doctors already practising a variety of manipulative techniques
and offering postgraduate teaching over eight weekends,
complemented by a follow-up weekend; more recently, its
President and Vice-President have been offering four-day
intensive courses to doctors. In 1986 it only had 300 members. Chiropractors, of course, dislike the idea of short
courses in manipulation, since they spend years of well-

supervised practice in developing the manual sensitivity to palpate the spine and carry out very specific, rather than generalized, adjustments. (In fact one or two GPs have recognized this and have taken, or are taking, the full AECC or MCS training.)

Where chiropractors would join forces with Dr Paterson, Vice-President of BAMM, however, is in his desire to make doctors much more aware of the importance of the spine. 'I'm not suggesting,' he says, 'that all doctors should be jumping about and thumping people. We want to sell the idea of manipulation to serious-minded doctors. I think they all ought to know, because of the incidence not only of drug dependency but of the side-effects of spinal problems like the common headache, chest pain and abdominal pain. Whether doctors do the manipulation themselves or not doesn't matter, provided they are aware, and that the people they refer them to have a training which makes them safe. There's nothing alternative about manipulation. We regard it as an extremely useful therapeutic option.'

Doctors may feel that they are already busy enough, without adding time-consuming techniques of adjustment to their services. In addition, manipulation requires a special gift for touch which not all doctors possess, or should be expected to. The more open-minded doctors, particularly the younger ones, recognize that they cannot be experts in everything, and do not feel professionally threatened by the existence of specialists who can succeed where they can't. Hopefully, this attitude is spreading, as expressed by Dr Drury: 'We quite welcome an alternative source of help for our patients. GPs are a fairly pragmatic group; if it works and if it helps, then scientific validation is not a side issue exactly, but is less relevant than the fact that the patient benefits ... The dividing line between alternative and professional is academic in a way; it's a shame it should be there at all.'

The Need for Research

For chiropractic to be incorporated into the NHS, pragmatism is not enough. Convincing individual doctors of the benefits of chiropractic is quite different from convincing medical and scientific authorities; for this, definitive, objective research is needed.

Research into any kind of therapy falls basically into two parts: scientific research, to show how the therapy works; and what has been dubbed 'consumer' research, to show how far it benefits people. With the former, chiropractic is confronted with a problem faced by other alternative therapies, which is a kind of medical double-think. As Research Director of the AECC, chiropractor Alan Breen is faced with the task of validating chiropractic. He points out – as does Dr Paterson and many others – that most medically prescribed drugs have not been scientifically validated or substantiated by clinical trial. (And although they have to be passed by the Committee of Safety on Medicines, many drugs, as we know, have later been found to be unsafe. It was not realized for some twenty years that the benzodiazepine group of tranquillizers were heavily addictive.) Yet practitioners of alternative therapies currently under government scrutiny, like homoeopathy and herbalism, are required to show not only that they are safe, but that they are effective, and why.

Apart from the area of pain relief, no one has established scientifically what happens during a manipulation and exactly how it benefits the patient, although – particularly since the 1960s – a considerable amount of research has been and is being done in chiropractic colleges all over the world, including the AECC.* Perhaps in time it will be

*For scientifically oriented readers, an up-to-date survey of research into chiropractic is provided in *The Chiropractic Theories, A Synopsis of Scientific Research* by Robert A. Leach, A.A., D.C., F.I.C.C., Williams & Wilkins, USA and London, 1986.

possible to show precisely what is going on inside the spine of a live patient at the time of an adjustment, and what effects this has on the nervous system.

There are other areas, besides back problems, where properly conducted research could be of enormous benefit: those involving Type O disorders. To quote *Chiropractic in New Zealand*, 'Chiropractors have for years been claiming that chiropractic treatment may be and in some cases is beneficial for [Type O disorders]. Yet it is astonishing to find that little if any constructive effort has been made by the medical profession to investigate these claims.' A few surveys have been carried out into the effects of manipulation on migraine, notably by a group at the University of New South Wales, at the instigation of the Australian government. These have not been well enough designed to give conclusive results, but patients treated by chiropractors and other manipulators were significantly improved when compared with others treated by mobilization. As mentioned earlier, research into the chiropractic treatment of colitis in infants is under way in Denmark, and there have been small studies among brain-damaged hyperactive children in the USA, again not sufficiently well designed to be medically acceptable. But if there is any possibility – and there seems no doubt as to the possibility – that chiropractic can improve these conditions, as well as asthma and others, it must deserve fuller investigation in the interests of patients. There is surely a case, for instance, for including chiropractic in the range of treatments offered for childhood asthma, even if it does not work for all; those for whom it *does* work would benefit enormously, and those for whom it does not would not be harmed by it.

Meanwhile, *how* something works seems less important in human terms than the fact that it does work, and can relieve suffering. You might think it would be relatively simple to tell whether a spinal adjustment, or series of adjustments, is beneficial to the patient with back pain.

Apparently it isn't. For some time now various researchers have been trying to set up research models with this object in view. *Back Pain*, published by the Office of Health Economics, refers to a review of fifty-nine trials of conservative therapies for low-back pain which 'revealed a widespread failure to adhere to the methodological and other criteria universally regarded as essential to a well-designed and valid investigation'.

What is 'a well-designed and valid investigation'? The 'double-blind controlled trial', which is widely regarded as scientifically acceptable when applied to drugs, is difficult to apply to manipulation. It involves two groups of patients, one receiving the drug and one receiving a placebo (a dummy pill); neither the patients nor the assessors of the trial know which group is which. Although efforts have been made at performing 'dummy' manipulations, it is difficult to pretend with any conviction to adjust someone's spine. In any case, as a pro-chiropractic doctor points out, the double-blind study is 'really treating people as though they were live rats, expecting that they would all have similar responses. That is the weakness of the medicine I'm trained in; it doesn't consider the individuality of the individual.' This is echoed by chiropractors like Stephen Carpenter: 'It's not until you start wanting to know about a particular complex metaphysical, psychological, chemical/mechanical animal, with his particular past, that you can really apply a treatment that's appropriate for that individual. That's why double-blind trials are so difficult. One person's back pain can have a totally different cause from another's.'

This difficulty affects research into all the alternative therapies, which are based on treating individuals as individuals; the Research Council for Complementary Medicine, formed in 1983, was set up to look into methods of researching alternatives which take such factors into account. Its autumn 1986 conference, 'The Patient as

Individual and Statistic', was concerned with precisely these questions.

Another huge problem in researching alternative therapies is the cost. Much medical research is funded by drug companies, who have no incentive to support therapies that are not drug-oriented. And to design and monitor scientifically valid trials requires input from experts. Alan Breen says: 'Chiropractors don't have the background to do good-quality scientific research by virtue of our education in chiropractic. Therefore the research that we need to do has to be always collaborative, with the help of people such as data managers, mathematicians, biochemists, physiologists, and so on, working as a team. But we need equipment, we need to be able to endow research fellowships, to educate ourselves, and all this costs money. I'd like to see more good training institutions in chiropractic, preferably in universities where you have the expertise. Researchers are very valuable because they stimulate and bring up the level of teaching in the undergraduate programme by being right at the forefront; it's not a question of just hammering the same old material, but of pushing it forward, which keeps the instructors on their toes.'

In Britain, a start at least was made in 1986, after a pilot test with fifty patients showed that a collaborative study between chiropractic and medicine was possible. The Medical Research Council's Epidemiology and Medical Care Unit at Northwick Park Hospital is cooperating with the BCA in running a randomized controlled trial with the aim of evaluating the reduction of disability in patients with low-back pain of mechanical origin. It is hoped to include 2,000 patients in all, at twelve different centres; half will be allocated at random to hospitals and half to chiropractic clinics. They will assess their own progress using postal questionnaires, on which the measures of outcome have been validated as reliable in previous medical trials. Funding has been something of a hold-up; the MRC has been able to provide £40,000, but £300,000 to £400,000 will be needed in all. It will therefore be some two or three years before results are available.

'There are other areas to be researched,' says Alan Breen, 'including pain, economics, and patient satisfaction, that won't be covered by this study. There is no single definitive study that is going to say yes or no to chiropractic. This will be an important one, though, because it will be scientifically valid, since it is set up in a very rigorous way. If you can make a scientifically valid statement it is very valuable.'

Obviously there are a number of possible outcomes for this research. But if chiropractic were shown to be clearly more effective than hospital treatment there would be a very strong case for its inclusion in the National Health Service, or for some other form of government recognition.

The Personal Touch

For chiropractic to be included in the NHS many details would have to be ironed out, including the differences, for example between AECC- and MCS-trained chiropractors. The BCA's unexplained rejection by the Professions Supplementary to Medicine was something of a slap in the face, since they fulfilled the PSM's main requirements. Nevertheless, some of its members were relieved. Joining the PSM would have made them subsidiary to doctors, and AECC chiropractors want their diagnostic abilities recognized as well as their manipulative skills. Even those who currently have good relationships with the medical profession complain that 'doctors don't like communicating with lesser mortals, they don't like being told a diagnosis that they themselves haven't organized'. One told me of a case in which a young patient suffered unnecessarily for some months. The chiropractor diagnosed an early bone growth, non-malignant but very painful, which he confirmed by X-ray. The orthopaedic surgeon with whom he was in touch initially rejected his diagnosis; three months (and some further unnecessary X-rays) later he acknowledged that it was in fact correct, and operated on the patient. With their specialist training BCA chiropractors feel they have a lot to offer medicine, and would like to be seen as equal but different partners with doctors, as dentists are. (McTimoney chiropractors would also welcome the opportunity to work within the NHS, again provided that they were able to keep their personal identity.)

There are other potential problems. Chiropractic is a numerically small profession; most chiropractors are fully employed as it is; would there be enough of them to meet NHS demands? Then there is the question of personal choice. The freedom of private practice means that patients can choose who will treat them. In the hospital system they are allocated to whoever is available. Dr Marcovitch says: 'There are doctors I wouldn't send patients to and others that I would and the same would go for alternative practitioners. There are some who I feel would be useful for certain things if not for others, and some I wouldn't touch with a barge pole. What I'm interested in is what a person's training has been, what their experience is and *what their motives are*. Then I could entrust a patient to them.' (The question of choice cuts both ways, of course; the private practitioner is in a privileged position compared with the GP who is obliged to treat all comers.)

If chiropractors were to be employed within the overworked hospital system, would they still be able to give the time, personal care and attention which are such valuable elements of their treatment? In the efforts to validate chiropractic scientifically, some chiropractors fear that the human and personal aspect may be forgotten: that, as with doctors, there may be a risk of over-emphasizing academic qualifications at the expense of a more spiritual or holistic approach, in which patient and healer are part of a mutual and cooperative process which allows healing to take place. The personal touch is something that scientific research does not take into account – indeed, it makes every effort to rule it out. For example, attempts at testing adjustments by reproducing them by machine is to ignore the scientifically unmeasurable magic that occurs when one human being lays caring hands on another. This is not to say that skill in adjustment is not important; it is. But behind every adjustment there is something less easily definable and testable: the chiropractor's unspoken attitude and beliefs,* his desire to heal, and his or her rapport with the patient. A McTimoney chiropractor says: 'Any student of anything, acupuncture, osteopathy or chiropractic, will tell you that when they're training and are being regularly treated by all and sundry they sometimes come out feeling horrific. It doesn't have much to do with whether you like the person or not, but whether they are the right person to treat you.' To maintain both freedom of choice and enough time for proper treatment, one answer might be for chiropractic and other forms of manipulation to be granted government recognition, as in other countries, so that patients could have their fees reimbursed by the state or by insurance schemes.

The Need to Pool Resources

In Britain there is so clearly a major gap in health care that, whatever the financial and logistical difficulties, urgent con-

---

*On the question of belief, the findings of Guy Lyon Playfair, author of *If This Be Magic* (Jonathan Cape, 1986), raise some interesting speculations as to the power of the *therapist*'s beliefs (not the patient's faith). Having studied the work of hypnotists who could cure patients of incurable diseases only so long as they didn't know they were incurable, Mr Playfair says: 'There is evidence to support the theory that the practitioner gets what he expects. If your GP believes in the pills he gives you, they will work; if he prescribes them to get rid of you, they won't.' I can't help wondering whether some of Palmer's 'miracle' cures came about because he didn't know they were impossible.

sideration should be given to providing skilled and expert treatment to all back sufferers at as early a stage as possible. It surely makes economic, let alone humanitarian, sense for back-pain sufferers to be treated before their problems become chronic. As Dr Marcovitch says, 'It would seem to me that it might be economic for the Health Service to contract for the services of people who have had a proper training and are on a register, or employ them on a part-time basis. Osteopathy and chiropractic could have a major role in the NHS. A major problem in the Health Service is enormous orthopaedic waiting-lists, enormous waiting times to be seen, enormous waiting times to be treated, and a service that's so snowed under that in fact it's going to provide no sort of service for certain things. For the majority of patients seen by orthopaedic surgeons, for example with low-back pain, there is no question of surgery and even diagnosis is very obscure. It seems to me there's a vast number of patients for whom there isn't really a service. But there are trained people to deal with those things, and it's a great pity we can't make use of them.'

The recognition of chiropractic in other countries has come about rather as a result of public pressure than of scientific proof. So far, the most convincing tests of its efficacy – in that they have led to positive action – have been those where assessment has been carried out by independent arbiters, neither doctors nor chiropractors. Firstly, there have been several studies carried out in the USA comparing chiropractic care with medical care, mainly by Workmen's Compensation Boards whose records were analysed by independent experts. Secondly, there was the New Zealand Commission of Inquiry into Chiropractic, in which an unbiased group consisting of a headmistress, a chemistry professor and a barrister heard and assessed evidence given on oath by chiropractors, doctors, physiotherapists and patients.

Although chiropractic in Britain has not suffered the

medical opposition described in *Chiropractic in New Zealand*, there does seem to be a sort of national negativity which makes it easier for us to find defects in each other rather than to look for the good – and this applies right across the board. It is not just the prejudiced doctor who will condemn all manipulation because he has come across one case of damage to a patient; the field of alternative therapies is itself divided into a multiplicity of different schools of thought and practice, who are all too inclined to criticize one another's work on similar grounds. It is understandable that people who have gone out on a limb to study for and work in an alternative profession feel justly proud of their own particular training and skills. It is a great pity when this leads them to discount the training and skills of others.

It is in the nature of the game that chiropractors, osteopaths and orthopaedic surgeons only see each other's failures. There are failures in every group. But for any one group to draw general conclusions from these without taking into account each other's successes is not only unscientific but a waste of time, energy and potential resources; as far as the public is concerned, criticism of the work of others tends to backfire on the criticizers rather than the criticized. The fact that there are choices in healing methods should enrich health care, not divide it. Individual therapists already recognize this. 'There is no right or wrong, there is what is right for you,' says a McTimoney chiropractor. And Victoria Cichy says: 'I think we are all involved in trying to get our message across to the medical profession, and also to the public. I don't see physiotherapists as being in competition with chiropractors and osteopaths; back pain is such a big problem.'

If the word 'holism' has any meaning other than as a currently popular catchword, it should imply wholeness and unity not just in the patient–therapist relationship but within the alternative professions themselves. Clearly, minimum standards of training need to be applied for the protection of patients, and a start was made in 1985 with the setting-up of the Council for Complementary and Alternative Medicine, of which the BCA is one of the eight founder members; the CCAM has elected to get together to work on the lengthy process of establishing standards. Once standards have been clarified the eventual membership of other groups, including the IPC, has not been ruled out.

The field of spinal manipulative therapy includes doctors who manipulate, physiotherapists, a variety of osteopathic schools and the two chiropractic schools; within these there are a multitude of techniques, approaches and levels of expertise. All of them have something to offer. The completion of this book coincided with the launch of the International Back Pain Society, formed at the instigation of Professor Michael Jayson, Professor of Rheumatology at the University of Manchester, with the intention of sharing the knowledge and experience of all professionals in this field. If the different disciplines can come together with open minds to pool their resources, they may present a powerful lobby for the promotion of manipulation first, and not as a last resort.

CARING FOR YOUR BACK

Chiropractors have a particular concern not only to do their best for their patient's problems, but to see that they don't recur. Patients can play an active part in their own cure and prevent future problems by following advice on exercise, body use, sitting, lifting, and so on, and by taking responsibility for themselves. As Bronwen Herbertson says, 'We use our "Rolls Royce" bodies like dodgem cars and feel very hard done by when they malfunction, even though we've taken less care of them in most cases than we would devote to a clapped-out mini-car.'

The value of seeing a chiropractor is that you will be given personal guidance to suit you as an individual. But here are some general guidelines for back sufferers, and for people who don't want to become back sufferers.

Be Aware!

If you live with mild aches and pains (which may or may not get worse in time) it is easy to become used to them and ignore them. In one way this is fine: I wouldn't suggest that everyone should become an instant hypochondriac – constantly worrying about pain can definitely make it worse. But pain is a warning signal, and it is sensible to pay attention to it by taking positive counter-action. You can make a start by noticing how you use your body in your daily activities.

Become aware of how you sit, stand, lie, and carry out tasks. Notice if you are tightening your neck and shoulder muscles unnecessarily, for example when reading, writing or telephoning, and learn to let them gently relax. Notice if any particular movements or postures aggravate back pain – and avoid them! You may find that some very simple adjustments to the way you do things will relieve tension and consequent pain. Simultaneously twisting while lifting or reaching out can be the last straw for a vulnerable disc; do you have to twist and reach out at the same time to get at your telephone or some other piece of equipment which could be moved to a more easily reachable place? Do you have to bend to get at papers or a filing-cabinet drawer? Notice how your kitchen shelves are arranged – do you have to bend and stretch more than is really necessary to reach items you use every day? See whether you can organize your environment to suit your back better.

Restoring the Balance

Many problems arise from the habit of using one side of the body more than the other, creating an imbalance and therefore vulnerability in the muscles around the spine. Examples are mothers who always carry the baby (or the shopping) on one side, lorry-drivers who always haul themselves into the cab with the same arm, typists who always twist to the left to read copy. Start noticing if you do any of these things, or regularly perform apparently unimportant actions one-sidedly, like always starting to climb the stairs with the same foot, or opening doors with the same hand. Notice whether you always stand with the weight on one leg. What happens when you transfer it to the other, or – preferably – allow the weight to fall equally on both? Help your body to re-balance by adopting the unhabitual hand, arm or leg, so that both sides are given an equal amount of use.

If you have been engaged in a one-sided activity – whether carrying heavy shopping or playing tennis –

there's a good re-balancing exercise taught at Touch for Health courses. Swing your right arm and left knee up, then your left knee and right arm, in a relaxed and regular fashion, so that you are doing a loose kind of marching on the spot. Keep it up for around six to twelve 'sets', or as long as feels comfortable. This is believed to balance the body's nervous and energy systems as well as the muscles, and can feel surprisingly refreshing.

Posture

Ideally, everyone needs personal advice on improving posture, as it's difficult for the individual to know what they are doing wrong and how to change it. A good chiropractor can help, of course. Many people swear by the Alexander

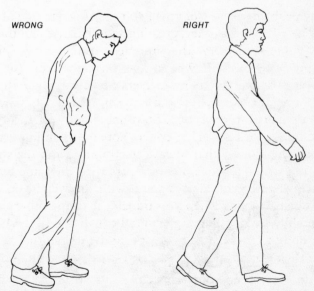

Slouching with rounded shoulders throws your spine out of balance. Walking tall makes you and your spine feel better

Technique, a method of re-educating the body not just in posture but in daily use. Some chiropractors recommend this, others are more dubious about it, but a number of people with back problems have found it helpful.

To improve your posture yourself, there are two extremes to avoid: one is slouching around with hunched shoulders and protruding stomach; the other is the chest-out, shoulders-back military stance, which can create an over-hollow back, and puts strains and tension in many places. Think of having a straight, upright spine, let your shoulders be relaxed and your tummy pulled in (without strain) and imagine your head floating upwards from the centre as if held up by an air balloon. When standing still, try to keep the weight equally on both feet.

Lordosis, an over-hollow back, is a common problem which can aggravate lower-back weakness and pain. Exercises to combat this are included in the 'Exercise' section below.

Lifting and Carrying

When lifting objects (or children) off the ground, bend your knees rather than your back, and let your legs do the lifting as you stand up; as mentioned above, avoid lifting and twisting at the same time. Apply the same principles to bed-making, particularly if the bed is low. Try to divide shopping or luggage into two loads so that you carry an equal weight on each side. Try to avoid lifting very heavy objects – that is, anything over about 10kg. This is sometimes easier said than done, but if you do have to lift something heavy, carry the weight in front of you rather than to the side, and keep your arms close in to your body which gives them added strength. Better still, keeping to these guidelines, get some help as well.

WRONG   RIGHT

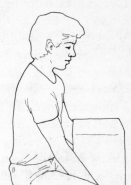

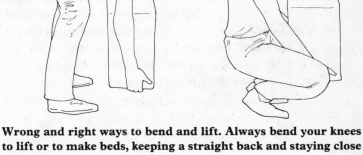

Wrong and right ways to bend and lift. Always bend your knees to lift or to make beds, keeping a straight back and staying close to whatever it is you are lifting

Sitting and Seating

Chiropractors tend to look at the body in engineering terms, and have done a good deal of research into problems of seating and furniture design. The views of some are beginning to be heard. For example, BCA chiropractor Dr Kim Jeffery advised the designer of the seats for British Rail's Advanced Passenger Train on the best support for the lumbar spine and on the correct position for headrests, after studying the profiles of 100 patients in his clinic.* And Ray Broome, Clinic Director of the AECC, was invited to address the firm of Mercedes-Benz in Germany after complaining to them that his new car had given him back-ache! They also fitted his car with a seat designed to his specifica-

* His work is described fully in two papers on the subject in the *European Journal of Chiropractic*, Vol. 32, 1984.

tions. Would that we could all receive such a service – but perhaps if more of us complained, more manufacturers would take notice.

Although things are slowly changing, much modern furniture design is positively bad for both posture and back problems, whether in offices, homes, public places or transport. Although human beings have grown an average of 10cm in height this century, furniture design has become 10cm lower! This encourages slouching, round shoulders, and a weakening of the lumbar area. So do our sedentary habits: after a day sitting at a desk many people – including, unfortunately, children – spend the evenings slumped in front of the television, creating weak spines for themselves.

So there are two steps to be taken: getting the right kind of furniture, and ensuring that you sit in it to your best advantage.

The working seat

For desk work of any kind the sitter should have the feet flat on the floor, and the body upright, tilted slightly forward. With a tilted seat the spine supports itself and does not need a backrest. The working surface should be below elbow level; for reading and writing a tilted surface is ideal (the Victorians knew what they were about with their sloping office desks!).

Anyone who has to sit for long hours at a desk is well advised to take regular breaks to stretch, get up and walk around, shrug or gently roll the shoulders, or do some gentle head-and-neck rolls. All these movements will help prevent the muscles and joints from becoming fixed and stressed.

For office furniture it is worth visiting a shop that specializes in back-conscious seating. Office chairs can now be bought with the requisite forward tilt, or (less expensively) an ordinary chair can be adapted simply by placing a triangular wedge on the seat (obtainable from a number of

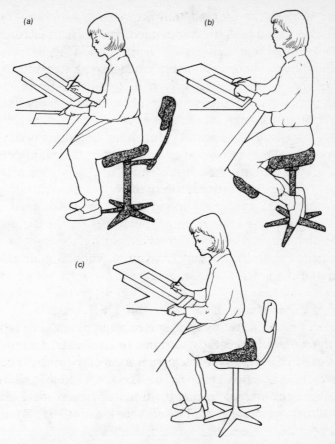

Are you sitting comfortably? Modern solutions to back strain at work include sloping work surfaces and forward-tilting seats to give lumbar support and keep the spine straight. Illustrated here are (a) the tilted office chair, (b) the Balans seat, and (c) a triangular wedge on the seat of an ordinary chair

suppliers, including Positive Posture, 120 Church Lane, London N2 0TB, telephone 01-883 7828/01-998 9997). The backless seats on which you rest your knees are good for keeping the spine upright and feel very comfortable when you try them out, but be warned – not all designs are ideal for long periods as they can compress the blood vessels in the knees. A number of suppliers are genuinely interested in providing suitable furniture and will give good advice on what to buy; these include Alternative Sitting, 17 Oxford Road, Abingdon, Oxon. OX14 2ED, telephone 0235 22777. Writing slopes are also obtainable from both firms mentioned above.

For travelling, a useful aid is an inflatable, shaped, low-back cushion which can be carried in the pocket. This is available from Sitco (South West) Ltd, 10 St Nicholas Road, Oxford OX4 4PP, telephone 0865 777 437.

Home seating

The ideal height for sofas and armchairs will depend on the height of the individual; however, many of them are much too low. As a not very tall person I was surprised to realize what a difference it made to my back when I raised the height of my sofa seat by adding an extra cushion. The seat depth from front to back should not exceed the length from the knee to the hip; over-deep seats are a very common design fault in sofas and easy chairs. You may think you are relaxing comfortably in one of these, but they cause the spine to curve unsupported just where it needs support, in the lower back. Requirements for orthopaedically comfortable living-room chairs, says Kim Jeffery, are:

1. Firm support low down in the back. If the chair back is only softly padded, you need firm padding near the bottom of the back. Most cushions are too soft for this; the support needs to be pretty solid – the consistency of a rolled-up towel.

2. The angle between the sloping back and the seat should be around 110°.

3. Unlike office seats, the squab (the part of the seat you sit on) should be tilted back 5–10 degrees, and most importantly, it should be cloth-covered. Wooden chairs may have

all the correct angles, but you will tend to slide forward when you sit on them.

Chiropractors, including Kim Jeffery, also recommend a seating aid which can be of benefit to anyone, but particularly to people in wheelchairs (notoriously bad for back support) or car-drivers. Called the Backfriend and made by the Liverpool firm of ME Design, it is a soft-covered seat back and squab, hinged so that it can be folded up and carried. It can, says Mr Jeffery, 'transform a rotten chair into a good one'. (It can be obtained by mail order from The Back Shop Mail Order Ltd, 24 New Cavendish Street, London W I M 7 L H; they stock other back aids such as back rests and air cushions.)

Driving seats

If you have back trouble, it is preferable not to drive at all. As cars have become sleeker and lower, Ray Broome points out, they are becoming less and less good for the back, forcing us to crouch forward or lean too far back, not only creating bad posture but adding to the general tension of driving. Bear this in mind when buying a new car; ideally, drivers should sit upright on a firmly padded seat with the spine well supported and legs comfortably extended; avoid over-soft seats. The top of the seat or headrest should be right behind the top of the head.

Beds

The ideal sleeping surface should be firm; soft mattresses give no support to the back. If your mattress is over-squashy, it can be remedied by placing a sheet of chipboard under it. At the same time, some 'orthopaedic' beds are over-hard, which can also create problems, since they do not yield to the contours of the body. So when buying a bed, look for a comfortably firm mattress and don't be shy of trying it out in the shop; also bear bed-making in mind, remembering that making a low bed can put a strain on the back.

Try to avoid too many pillows, which can strain the neck and cause headaches. Conversely, people with low-back pain may find this eased by sleeping on their sides with a pillow between their knees and a second one tucked into the back.

While on the subject of beds, low-back pain can be a blight to one's sex life. For women with low-back pain, particularly if they have heavy partners, the 'missionary position' is far from ideal. Whichever partner has backache, it needn't upset the relationship if you experiment together to find the most enjoyable positions. It could even be fun!

Exercise

One reason backs are such a problem today is lack of exercise. Regular, gentle exercise is good for everyone, and for the health of the whole body. If you are actually undergoing treatment for your back, be advised by your chiropractor or doctor; during a course of treatments he or she may advise you to rest rather than exercise, particularly at the beginning while your body is still in the process of adjusting. Some exercises may be inadvisable for your condition. Remember that pain is a warning sign, and performing movements that hurt (with all deference to Jane Fonda) is unlikely to be good for you.

One of the very best exercises for backs is walking, which costs nothing and is an excellent stress-reliever. Jogging and running are good for the already fit, but can over-stress backs, knees and ankles if there is any weakness; even for the fit it appears that jogging on hard surfaces can produce some problems. There's a lot of opportunity these days for exercising at aerobics classes, gyms and fitness centres, but instruction can be variable in quality. I was shocked at the posture of some of the women at an aerobics class I visited once only! The instructress made no attempt to correct it, nor did she get participants to check their heart-rate by taking their pulse, as is generally recommended; in fact the aim seemed to be to put as much strain on the body as possible!

There are also some excellent classes around as well, with instructors well trained in anatomy who pay individual attention to members. In any class the quality of instruction is at least as important as the type of exercise. So while yoga, dance, keep fit, weight-lifting, and so on, can be excellent for the back, posture and general health, don't commit yourself to a class without checking it out first, and always tell the instructor if you have a back problem; a good instructor will bear this in mind and warn you about movements that are not appropriate for you. Some types of movement like Medau and T'ai Chi are particularly good for posture, balance, relaxation and flexibility.

Swimming can be good, but if you do the wrong stroke for your type of back it can be disastrous, as we have seen! Both butterfly and breast-stroke hollow the back, which is not good if there is a lumbar weakness. Swimming on the back is best, whether backstroke or an inverted breast-stroke. Make sure you don't stay wet and cold afterwards.

Below are some general exercises for strengthening the back and preventing problems. If you are currently having treatment, check with your chiropractor or doctor before you embark on them.

Exercises

Preparation

Wear loose, comfortable clothing. Before an exercise session, allow yourself a 'warm-up period' of gentle stretching to allow the muscles to loosen up; a warm bath can also ease tense muscles beforehand. Start the movements slowly and gently, and don't overdo them. Do, however, exercise regularly.

A. Exercises for strengthening the lower back and combating lordosis (hollow back)

Start by performing each of the following contractions for 3 to 5 seconds at a time, adding 1 second each week and stopping at a maximum of 12 seconds. Repeat each exercise up to five times in any one session. For floor exercises, choose a carpeted surface.

1. PLIÉS: Stand with feet hip-width apart, pointing forward. Bend the knees slightly, tighten the buttocks and pull in the stomach muscles so that the pelvis is tucked under. Hold for a few seconds. (This can be done at intervals during the day, while you're telephoning, washing-up, or waiting in a queue. Practised regularly it also does wonders for the stomach and waistline, and tightens thigh muscles.)

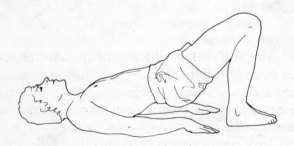

2. PELVIC TILT: Lie on your back on the floor with feet hip-width apart and knees raised. Breathing out, tighten your stomach muscles, thighs and buttocks, lifting your hips off the floor. Breathing in, gently lower hips to the floor and relax.

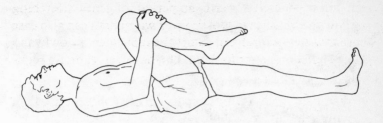

3. KNEE-PULLS: Lie flat on the floor. Bring one knee to-wards your chest, clasp your hands around it and pull it firmly towards you, at the same time keeping the other leg firmly stretched. Hold, release and gently lower leg to floor; repeat with the other leg.

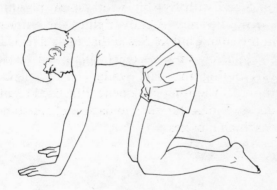

4. CAT-ARCH: Kneel on all fours on the floor. Check that your body is equally balanced on both sides by looking at the arch made by your legs (you may be surprised to see that what feels even is actually not). Breathing out and contracting the stomach muscles, push the centre of your back upwards. Follow this by lowering your buttocks on to your heels and your forehead on to the floor, with your hands still on the floor and arms out-stretched in a 'praying' position. Breathe gently into your back, allowing it to open out and release tension.

5. FLATTENING A HOLLOW BACK: Stand in a doorway

(30″–36″ wide) with your back and head flat against one side of the door jamb. Lift one leg and place the foot on the opposite side of the doorway. Breathe in and push hard. Repeat with the other foot.

6. THIGH CONTRACTION: Take an object about 16″ in diameter, such as a wastepaper basket. Sit on the floor with legs stretched out straight, and put the object between your feet, if necessary putting your hands on the floor behind you for balance. Breathing in, squeeze the legs together hard against the object. This helps to firm the inner thigh.

B. Exercises for the neck and upper back

As with lower-back exercises, do these gently at first, and don't force them if they cause pain. Start by repeating each three to five times, building this up as you gain strength and flexibility. These are good to do during the day if you are stuck at a typewriter or word-processor.

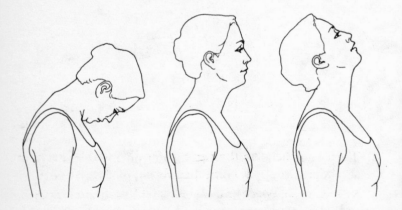

1. Tuck in your chin and gently bend the head forward, trying to touch your chin to your chest; hold, then bend the head backwards as far as it will comfortably go.

2. Bend the head to one side, as if to touch your shoulder

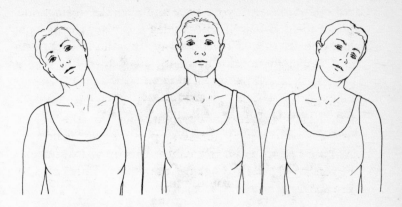

with your ear; keep your head facing forward. Repeat on the other side.

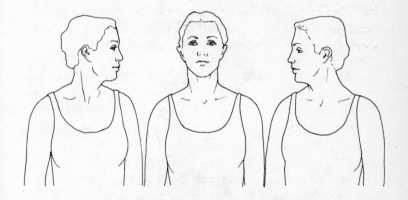

3. Turn your head to the right as far as possible, keeping shoulders dropped; hold, then repeat on the left.

4. Roll your neck and head in small circles, first clockwise, then anti-clockwise. Let the circles expand, but don't force the neck to stretch. Keep the movement loose and comfortable.

5. Shrug your shoulders up to your ears, hold, then let them drop free and relaxed.

Relaxation

Many people feel guilty if they take time out to 'do nothing'. Yet regular relaxation sessions can reduce pain, relieve mental tension and encourage the body's own self-healing process. So don't regard relaxing as doing nothing, but as a powerful form of self-help.

Relaxation is extremely simple, but many of us find it hard to do. Aids include some good relaxation classes run at evening institutes and fitness centres, and a variety of audio tapes. But try this basic routine for ten to twenty minutes daily. Decide beforehand that during this period you will set aside work or worries, take the phone off the hook and, if you like, put on some soothing music.

Lie on the floor, with a small cushion under your head if you prefer. People with low-back pain may also find it more comfortable to place a cushion under the knees. Start by taking a deep breath and stretching the whole body taut – arms, legs, fingers, toes, and even your facial muscles. Breathe out and let everything go. Repeat this stretch-and-let-go two or three times.

Now pay attention to your breathing. Place your hands on your midriff and notice whether your breath is moving your upper chest or your abdomen. Allow your breathing to expand your lower rib cage and abdomen, and – without forcing – let it become deeper. Keep your hands on your diaphragm, or place them by your sides, whichever is the most comfortable. Then, with your attention placed lightly on your breathing, simply allow your body to be at rest, letting everything go, sinking into the floor, until you are deeply relaxed. Notice any areas of pain in your body and try to relax into them rather than tensing up against them.

If you find it hard to let go completely, use your imagination as an extra aid. For example, visualize your body as a sandbag, with sand trickling out at the seams. Or imagine that you are floating in the sea, breathing in rhythm with the gentle waves. Or visualize your tension leaving you as you breathe out, and health and energy coming into your system with each in-breath. Alternatively, if visualization doesn't appeal to you, repeat to yourself silently a soothing word such as 'peace' or 'harmony' as you breathe in and out.

At the end of a relaxation session stretch again and always get up slowly. Once you have acquired the art of letting go, you will find it easy to do at fraught times during the day.

A Positive Attitude

The mind can have a tremendously strong influence on the body. There are good biochemical reasons for this, as medicine has recently been discovering, though there is still a lot more to be learned about the exact processes by which our thoughts affect all our physical processes. So adopting and maintaining a positive attitude towards one's health can be a strong contributive factor in the healing process. Just as an experiment, try sitting for two minutes while telling yourself that you feel terrible – but please don't make a habit of it, and don't do it at a time when you are feeling low to start with; treat it as a scientific test! Spend the next five minutes telling yourself you feel well, happy, and confident of the future (by all means make a habit of this). Notice how your body feels after each session. Notice, too, that you have a choice of what to think and feel. Positive thoughts really can encourage healing.

Diet

A healthy, balanced diet can be an important factor in back care. For example, both over-weight and constipation can

exacerbate back pain; if either of these is a problem, seek
advice from your chiropractor or doctor or a nutritionist. In
addition, some foods and drinks, like red meat, white flour,
sugar, coffee and alcohol, seem to aggravate muscular pains
(and in certain diseases like rheumatoid arthritis they are
a contributory factor in some cases). As with your daily
activities, it pays to become aware of what particular foods
or drinks do to you – for example, red wine, or even in some
instances tap-water, may exacerbate pain in some people,
though not all; they may not realize it until they start taking
notice. If you are in doubt about your diet, it could be
worth consulting a reputable nutritionist, naturopath or
medical herbalist. General dietary guidelines for back sufferers are similar to those widely advocated these days for
over-all health. If you follow them, constipation shouldn't
be a problem, by the way!

Eat plenty of fresh fruits, salads and vegetables, and
plenty of fibre-containing foods (whole grains like brown
rice, wholemeal bread and pasta, and pulses like beans and
lentils). Avoid red meats, fatty meats (particularly sausages
and salamis which also contain preservatives) and fried
foods, processed foods, sugar, sweets and white flour. Eat
cheese and other dairy products in moderation only; for
protein go for low-fat cheeses, chicken, fish and nuts. Drink
tea and coffee only in moderation, and experiment with
herbal teas which can do your system positive good.

Further Reading

Since there is not the space here to go fully into all aspects
of back care, the following books are recommended for
readers who want to know more and do more for themselves.

Diets to Help Arthritis by Helen MacFarlane, Thorson's
   Publishers, Wellingborough, 1979

A Doctor's Proven New Home Cure for Arthritis by Giraud W. Campbell, D.O., Thorson's Publishers, Wellingborough, 1979. (Includes diet, exercises and positive thinking)

Let's Get Well and other titles by Adelle Davis, Unwin Paperbacks, London, 1974. (Still the classics in healthy eating)

Rheumatism and Arthritis by Malcolm I. V. Jayson and Allan St J. Dixon, Pan Books, London, 1984

The Back: Relief from Pain by Dr Alan Stoddard, Martin Dunitz, London, 1979. (Covers exercises, body use/posture, but not diet)

To find a chiropractor: see under British Chiropractic Association, European Chiropractors' Union, Institute of Pure Chiropractic, etc., below.

Chiropractic Organizations

BRITAIN

The Anglo-European College of Chiropractic, Parkwood Road, Bournemouth BH5 2DF. Telephone 0202 431021

The British Chiropractic Association, 5 First Avenue, Chelmsford, Essex CM1 1RX. Telephone 0245 358487. (For copy of register, write enclosing a 9″ × 6½″ s.a.e.)

The Chiropractic Advancement Association, Honorary Secretary: Mrs Betty Kenny, 38a Upper Richmond Road West, East Sheen, London SW14 8DD. Telephone 01-878 3989

The Institute of Pure Chiropractic, P.O. Box 126, Oxford OX1 1UF. Telephone 0865 246687. (For copy of register, write enclosing a 9″ × 4½″ s.a.e.)

The McTimoney Chiropractic School, P.O. Box 127, Oxford OX1 1HH. Telephone 0865 246786

AUSTRALIA

Australian Chiropractors Association, Federal Secretariat, Executive Director: Dr J. A. Sweaney, 1 Martin Place, Linden, NSW 2778. Telephone (047) 53 1013

Philip Institute of Technology, Head, School of Chiropractic: A. M. Kleynhans, D.C., Plenty Road, Bundoora, Victoria 3083

CANADA

Canadian Chiropractic Association, Executive Director: J. L. Watkins, D.C., and Canadian Memorial College, President: I. D. Coulter, Ph.D., both at 1900 Bayview Avenue, Toronto, Ontario M4 3E6

EUROPE

The European Chiropractors' Union, Secretary: Dr A. Metcalfe, 19 Strawberry Hill Road, Twickenham, Middx. TW1 4QB. Telephone 01-891 6158

Non-British national members of the ECU (1986) are as follows: Belgium, Denmark, Finland, France, West Germany, Greece, Italy, Netherlands, Norway, Spain, Sweden, Switzerland. Names and addresses of chiropractors in any of these countries can be obtained by writing to the Secretary at the above address; a complete register of members can also be obtained from him on request, enclosing a 9″ × 6½″ s.a.e. (stamped for up to 100g).

HONG KONG

Hong Kong Chiropractors Association, 27 Cameron Road, 3/F Tsimshatsui, Kowloon, Hong Kong

JAPAN

Japanese Chiropractors Association, 5–9, 3-Chome, Kita-Aoyama, Minato-Ku, Tokyo 107. Telephone 03 478 2713

NEW ZEALAND

New Zealand Chiropractors Association, P.O. Box 2858, Wellington. Telephone 04 72 1716

SOUTH AFRICA

The Chiropractic Association of South Africa, 701 Poynton House, Gardiner Street, Durban 4001, Natal

UNITED STATES OF AMERICA

American Chiropractic Association, 1916 Wilson Boulevard, Arlington, VA 22201. Telephone 703 276 8800

International Chiropractors Association, 1901 L Street NW, Suite 800, Washington D.C. 20036. Telephone 202 659 6476

Other Organizations Mentioned

The Back Pain Association, Grundy House, 31–33 Park Road, Teddington, Middx. TW11 0AB. Telephone 01-977 5474/5

The British Association of Manipulative Medicine, 14 Wimpole Street, London W1M 7AB

The British Touch for Health Association, 29 Bushey Close, High Wycombe, Bucks. HP12 3HL. Telephone 0494 37409

Council for Complementary and Alternative Medicine, Suite 1, 19a Cavendish Square, London W1M 9AD. Telephone 01-409 1440

International Back Pain Society, Secretariat, Howletts Lane, Ruislip, Middx. HA4 7RS. Telephone 01-206 1511

Research Council for Complementary Medicine, Suite 1, 19a Cavendish Square, London W1M 9AD. Telephone 01-493 6930

International College of Applied Kinesiology, P.O. Box 680547, Park City, Utah 84068, USA

BIBLIOGRAPHY

Bach, Marcus, *The Chiropractic Story*, Si-Nel Publishing, Georgia, USA, 1986

Bourdillon, J. F., F.R.C.S., *Spinal Manipulation*, 3rd edition, William Heinemann Medical Books Ltd, London, and Appleton-Century-Crofts, New York, 1985

British Medical Association, *Alternative Therapy*, BMA, London, 1986

Campbell, Giraud W., D.O., *A Doctor's Proven New Home Cure for Arthritis*, Thorson's Publishers, Wellingborough, 1983

Commission of Inquiry into Chiropractic, *Chiropractic in New Zealand*, Hasselberg (Government Printer), Wellington, NZ, 1979

Complementary Medical Research, ed. Hugh L'Etang, Vol. I, 1, RCCM, London, 1986

Consumers' Association, *Avoiding Back Trouble*, Consumer Publications, London, 1978

Delvin, Dr David, *You and Your Back*, revised edition, Pan Books, London, 1977

Department of Health and Social Security, *Working Group on Back Pain*, Report to the Secretary of State for Social Services and Secretary of State for Scotland, HMSO, London, 1979

Dintenfass, Dr Julius, *Chiropractic: A Modern Way to Health*, Pyramid Books, New York, 1966

Eagle, Robert, *Alternative Medicine: A Guide to the Medical Underground*, Futura Publications, London, 1978

European Journal of Chiropractic, ed. R. Molloy, Vol. 33, Nos. 1 and 4, Blackwell Scientific Publications, Oxford, 1985

Fraser, John Lloyd, *The Medicine Men: A Guide to Natural Medicine*, Thames/Methuen, London, 1981

Fulder, Stephen, M.A., Ph.D., *The Handbook of Complementary Medicine*, Coronet Books, London, 1984

Haldeman, Scott, D.C., Ph.D., M.D., ed., *Modern Developments in the Principles and Practice of Chiropractic*, Appleton-Century-Crofts, New York, 1980

Hall, Hamilton, M.D., *Be Your Own Back Doctor*, Granada Publishing, London, 1983

Hulke, Malcolm, *The Encyclopedia of Alternative Medicine and Self-Help*, Rider & Co., London, 1978

Inglis, Brian, *Fringe Medicine*, Faber and Faber, London, 1964

Inglis, Brian, *Natural Medicine*, Fontana/Collins, London, 1979/80

Inglis, Brian, and West, Ruth, *The Alternative Health Guide*, Michael Joseph, London, 1983

Jayson, Malcolm I. V., *Back Pain: The Facts*, Oxford University Press, Oxford/New York/Toronto, 1981

Leach, Robert A., *The Chiropractic Theories: A Synopsis of Scientific Research*, revised edition, Williams & Wilkins, Baltimore/London/Los Angeles/Sydney, 1986

McClusky, Thorp, *Your Health and Chiropractic*, 2nd edition, Pyramid Books, New York, 1964

Maitland, G. D., *Vertebral Manipulation*, 3rd edition, Butterworths, London, 1973

Melzack, Ronald, *The Puzzle of Pain*, Penguin Books, Harmondsworth, 1973

Office of Health Economics, *Back Pain*, OHE, London, 1985

Palmer, D. D., *The Chiropractor*, Los Angeles, 1914, republished by Health Research, California, 1970

Palmer, David D., B.S., D.C., *Three Generations: A Brief History of Chiropractic*, Palmer College of Chiropractic, Davenport, Iowa, 1967

Paterson, John K., M.B., B.S., M.R.C.G.P., and Burn, Loic, B.A., M.R.C.S., L.R.C.P., D.Phys.Med., *An Introduction to Medical Manipulation*, MTP Press, Lancaster, and Hingham, USA, 1985

Rush, Anne Kent, *The Basic Back Book*, Wildwood House, London, 1980

Schafer, R. C., D.C. (ed.), *Chiropractic Health Care*, 2nd edition, Foundation for Chiropractic Education and Research, Iowa, 1977

Scofield, Arthur G., D.C., *Chiropractice: The Science of Specific Spinal Adjustment*, 2nd edition, Thorson's Publishers, Wellingborough, 1981

Sportelli, Louis, D.C., *Introduction to Chiropractic*, 8th edition, Palmerton, Pa., 1986

Stanway, Dr Andrew, *Alternative Medicine: A Guide to Natural Therapies*, Penguin Books, Harmondsworth, 1979

Stierwalt, Dr D. D., *Adjusting the Child*, Stierwalt, USA, 1976

Stoddard, Alan, M.D., *The Back: Relief from Pain*, Martin Dunitz, London, 1979

Valentine, Tom and Carole, *Applied Kinesiology*, Thorson's Publishers, Wellingborough and New York, 1985

Wainwright, Denys, M.B., N.Ch.Orth., F.R.C.S., D.Sc. (Hon.), *Arthritis and Rheumatism: What they are – What you can do to help yourself*, Paperfronts, Elliot Right Way Books, Kingswood, 1982

Weiant, C. W., D.C., Ph.D., and Goldschmidt, S., D.C., *Medicine and Chiropractic*, New York, 1966

Wilk, Chester A., D.C., *Chiropractic Speaks Out*, Wilk Publishing Co., Illinois, 1983

INDEX